Dearest Yueshi,

Chocolate for Your Soul

May you build happy and
meaningful moments here in
Seattle, WA.

Love,
Ai Lin
Sep 28, 2022

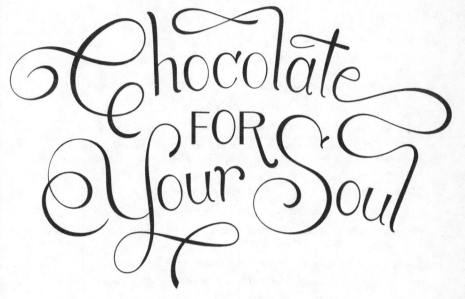

Chocolate FOR Your Soul

*Food, faith, and fun to satisfy your
deepest craving*

SHERI ROSE SHEPHERD

Bestselling author of the His Princess™ series

TYNDALE®
MOMENTUM

An Imprint of Tyndale House Publishers, Inc.

Visit Tyndale online at www.tyndale.com.

Visit Tyndale Momentum online at www.tyndalemomentum.com.

Visit Sheri Rose Shepherd at hisprincess.com.

Tyndale Momentum and the Tyndale Momentum logo are registered trademarks of Tyndale House Publishers, Inc. Tyndale Momentum is an imprint of Tyndale House Publishers, Inc., Carol Stream, Illinois.

Chocolate for Your Soul: Food, Faith, and Fun to Satisfy Your Deepest Craving

Previously published in 2012 as *If You Have a Craving, I Have a Cure* by Tyndale House Publishers under ISBN 978-1-4143-6692-0

Designed by Jennifer Phelps

Published in association with the Loyal Arts Literacy Agency, PO Box 1414, Bend, OR 97709.

Scripture quotations are taken from the *Holy Bible*, New Living Translation, copyright © 1996, 2004, 2015 by Tyndale House Foundation. Used by permission of Tyndale House Publishers, Inc., Carol Stream, Illinois 60188. All rights reserved.

Library of Congress Cataloging-in-Publication Data

Names: Shepherd, Sheri Rose, date, author.
Title: Chocolate for your soul : refreshing your relationship with God
   through food, faith, and fun / Sheri Rose Shepherd.
Other titles: If you have a craving, I have a cure
Description: Carol Stream, IL : Tyndale House Publishers, Inc., 2016. |
   Previous edition: If you have a craving, I have a cure. Carol Stream, Ill.
   : Tyndale Momentum, c2012. | Includes index.
Identifiers: LCCN 2016011147 | ISBN 9781496413499 (sc : alk. paper)
Subjects: LCSH: Food--Religious aspects--Christianity. | Dinners and
   dining—Religious aspects—Christianity.
Classification: LCC BR115.N87 S54 2016 | DDC 241/.68—dc23 LC record available at
   http://lccn.loc.gov/2016011147

Printed in the United States of America

22   21   20   19   18   17   16
 7   6   5   4   3   2   1

I would like to dedicate this book to my beautiful girls . . .

My Daughter
Emmy Joy Shepherd

My Daughter-in-Love
Amanda Shepherd

My Granddaughter
Olive True Shepherd

My Spiritual Daughter
Julia Jacobo

Contents

Introduction

Chocolate for Your Soul

*Taste and see that the LORD is good. Oh, the joys
of those who take refuge in him!*

PSALM 34:8

ASK WOMEN TO NAME their guilty pleasures or biggest cravings, and chocolate is likely to be on the list. After all, most of us find its sweet, creamy texture both soothing and delicious. No wonder chocolate is a staple in our pantries and a common treat at women's gab groups. Interestingly, science has discovered that cacao, the natural base of chocolate, provides many health benefits. For instance, eating chocolate stimulates the release of endorphins, chemicals in the brain that lead to feelings of happiness and pleasure. Dark chocolate may also help lower blood pressure and improve the cardiovascular system.

This sweet treat may be good for your heart, but God invites you to indulge in blessings that are like chocolate for your soul. He offers you three amazing gifts—food, faith, and fun—to satisfy and refresh you and your loved ones. Much as we crave chocolate, He wants us to desire more of Him and His good gifts.

Life can be hard, so it is sometimes tempting to focus on what you are not allowed to do and what you should not eat, but that will leave you feeling deprived and depressed, bored and burned out. That's not how God intends for you to live. It's time to let go of guilt, grab hold of grace, recapture the life God made you for, and then . . . *live it*!

In this book I will share many of the benefits and blessings of following Christ as you discover a new kind of faith walk, one filled with joy and a refreshing perspective on life. I'm also excited to share with you some delicious, healthy recipes that helped me conquer chronic fatigue and lose over fifty pounds and keep it off. (For some delicious dishes featuring chocolate, see chapter 1. And for even more faith and food coaching via video, visit hisprincess.com.)

Together you and I will learn to embrace the life Christ wants us to live while enjoying the wholesome and amazing food our God created for us. (Please note: I am not a medical professional, so if you are looking to make lasting changes to your diet or other parts of your health regimen, be sure to check with your doctor first, particularly if you have any medical conditions.)

As the wisest man who ever ruled, King Solomon, said in Ecclesiastes 5:18:

It is good for people to eat, drink, and enjoy their work under the sun during the short life God has given them, and to accept their lot in life.

You are about to taste and see that the Lord is good and that your faith can become a fulfilling adventure. That's great for the soul!

Love,
Sheri Rose
hisprincess.com

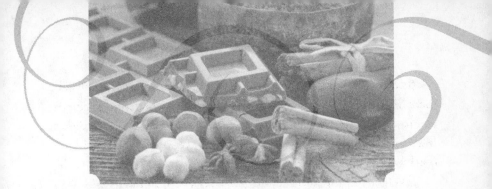

CHAPTER 1

Craving Something Rich

Chocolate Recipe Relief and Treasured Faith

I AM CONVINCED that chocolate should be in the food pyramid underneath fruits and vegetables. I often wonder if there will be unlimited chocolate fountains flowing in heaven (preferably the kind of chocolate that does not cause migraines). I believe chocolate is a gift from God, and believe me, in this chapter I think you're going to find some relief from the guilt you feel for craving it.

Soul Food

And I will give you treasures hidden in the darkness—secret riches. I will do this so you may know that I am the LORD, the God of Israel, the one who calls you by name.

ISAIAH 45:3

God's Word tells us that wherever our treasure is, there our heart will be also. Many times we miss the secret treasures the Lord desires to give us, because our hearts are so focused on what we want. As a result, we miss the better and richer life God designed for us.

Let's look at those riches that will last forever and crave everlasting wealth. When we do, we will leave a rich legacy for all those we love and know. After all, we brought nothing into this world, and we will leave with nothing except a rich faith and treasure in heaven.

New Life Recipes
. . . .

1. LIVE AS ROYALTY

For you are a chosen people. You are royal priests, a holy nation, God's very own possession. . . . He called you out of the darkness into his wonderful light.

I PETER 2:9

Live like a chosen child of the King. In other words, talk more about your riches in heaven and the blessings of being God's chosen one than about your burdens here on earth.

To remind you of your "royal status," you might frame one of your favorite Scriptures or eat rich dark chocolate while reading His Word in the evening.

2. INVEST IN ETERNITY

They themselves will be wealthy, and their good deeds will last forever.

PSALM 112:3

Make it your goal to do one thing a week that has eternal value. Give money to a great cause or e-mail words of encouragement to a friend. Commit to pray one day a week for our country.

3. COUNT THE COST

What do you benefit if you gain the whole world but are yourself lost or destroyed?

LUKE 9:25

Take a few moments to make a list of what you do with your time and energy each day. Next to this list, jot down the names of people you hang out with, what good is coming from those relationships, and what results (what the Bible calls "fruit") you are seeing from the ways you spend your time. Then pray and ask God to show you if these activities are all worth investing in.

POWER UP WITH PRAYER

Dear friend, I hope all is well with you and that you are as healthy in body as you are strong in spirit.

3 JOHN 1:2

*Dear God,
I want to live a rich life that will leave a legacy, so please give me what I need to have a rich faith. Give me as much as You want to provide for me and to help meet the needs of others, but not so much that I forget to rely on You.
Amen.*

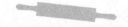

FOOD TRUTH

No food . . . is richer than becoming a reflection of His glory.

Real Rich Recipes

Sometimes, particularly on special occasions like birthdays and anniversaries, nothing is more appropriate than chocolate or a special cake. Indulge your sweet spot with one of these delicious recipes.

ALMOND CHOCOLATE SMOOTHIE
Serves 2–3

Ingredients:

1 cup almond milk

1 cup chocolate Rice Dream ice cream
    (or low-fat chocolate ice cream)

1 teaspoon honey

1 teaspoon almond extract

1–2 cups ice

Directions:

1. Mix all ingredients together in a blender until smooth.
2. Pour into glasses and enjoy!

Recipe tip:

You can use real almonds instead of almond extract to make this more of a raw recipe.

CRAVING CHOCOLATE CAKE

Serves 12

Ingredients:

1 package Pamela's chocolate cake mix or another gluten-free
    cake mix

1 package Pamela's dark chocolate frosting mix (optional)

1 cup sour cream

1 cup canola oil

4 eggs

½ cup warm water

2 cups semisweet chocolate chips

Powdered sugar, if desired

Pint of fresh raspberries, if desired

Directions:

1. Preheat oven to 350°.
2. In a large bowl, mix together the cake and frosting mix (if
   added), sour cream, oil, eggs, and water. Stir in the chocolate
   chips, and pour batter into a well-greased, 12-cup Bundt pan.
3. Bake for 50–55 minutes, or until a wooden toothpick inserted
   comes out clean.
4. Cool cake thoroughly in pan at least an hour and a half before
   inverting onto a plate. If desired, dust the cake with powdered
   sugar and place a few raspberries alongside each piece.

Recipe tip:

*After making the cake, cut it up in small slices; seal each in
Tupperware and freeze so you can use individual slices as
needed.*

CAROB PUDDING

Serves 2–4

Ingredients:

2 avocados

1 cup honey

¼ cup carob powder or unsweetened dark cocoa powder

¼ cup cocoa powder

1 tablespoon raw sugar or stevia

Directions:

In a blender, mix all ingredients until mixture is smooth and creamy. Add water as needed for desired consistency.

Recipe tip:

Add semisweet chocolate chips for a chocolaty surprise in the pudding. This pudding will keep for three days in the fridge.

CHOCOLATE DIP

Fills a small-size bowl

Ingredients:

½ cup unsweetened dark cocoa powder

½ cup honey or agave syrup

1 teaspoon vanilla extract

Directions:

Place all ingredients in blender and mix until smooth.

Recipe tip:

You can heat this up if you want your chocolate dipping sauce warm. Make sure to have your favorite fruit cut and ready to dip and enjoy!

MAKE MINE CHOCOLATE CAKE
Serves 12

Ingredients:

1¾ cups whole-grain or gluten-free flour

2 cups sugar

¾ cup unsweetened dark cocoa powder

2 teaspoons baking soda

1 teaspoon baking powder

1 teaspoon sea salt

1 tablespoon instant coffee (optional)

2 eggs

1 cup buttermilk

½ cup canola oil

1 teaspoon vanilla extract

Directions:

1. Preheat oven to 350°.
2. Grease and flour two 9-inch round cake pans or one 9 x 13-inch pan.
3. In a large bowl, combine flour, sugar, cocoa, baking soda, baking powder, salt, and instant coffee, if desired. Make a well in the center.
4. Add eggs, buttermilk, oil, and vanilla. Beat for 2 minutes on medium speed. Batter will be thin. Pour into prepared pans.
5. Bake for 30 to 40 minutes, or until toothpick inserted in center of cake comes out clean.
6. Cool for 10 minutes, then remove from pans and finish cooling on a wire rack. Layer and frost as desired.

Recipe tip:
Use the Chocolate Dip recipe on page 169 as frosting for this cake.

PURE FUDGE LOVE
Serves 24

Ingredients:

9.7-ounce bar of semisweet chocolate

3 cups raw sugar

¾ cup unsalted butter

⅔ cup unsweetened coconut milk

7 ounces marshmallow creme

2 teaspoons vanilla extract

Directions:

1. Butter a 9 x 13-inch baking dish or line it with parchment paper.
2. Chop the chocolate bar fine, and set it aside.
3. Place the sugar, butter, and coconut milk in a thick-bottomed, medium-large saucepan. Slowly bring the mixture to an active boil, stirring constantly. Continue boiling for five minutes over medium heat. If you are using a candy thermometer, it should read about 235°.
4. Remove from heat, and stir in the chopped chocolate. Continue stirring until the chocolate is melted. Then add the marshmallow creme and vanilla.
5. Pour the fudge mixture into the prepared baking dish, and let it cool.

Recipe tip:

You can also use this as a hot fudge chocolate dip!

SHAKIN' ME TO PIECES SMOOTHIE
Serves 2–3

Ingredients:

¾ cup peanut butter

3 cups ice (more if needed)

3 cups chocolate almond milk

1 tablespoon raw sugar or stevia

¼ cup semisweet chocolate chips

½ cup chocolate protein powder

Directions:

Place all ingredients in blender and mix for 1 to 2 minutes, until smooth. Pour and enjoy!

Recipe tip:

If you are allergic to peanuts, try using almond or cashew butter instead.

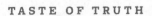

TASTE OF TRUTH

**No amount of riches can buy you
peace of mind or a home in heaven.**

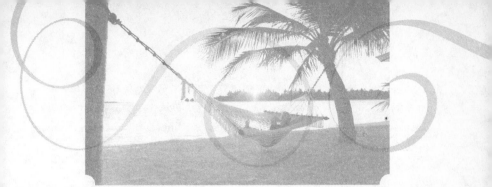

CHAPTER 2

Craving Rest and Relaxation

Healthy Comfort Food and Recipes for Rest

WHEN MY DAUGHTER WAS A TODDLER, she never wanted to take a nap. No matter what I did to make naptime appealing, she refused to lie down without a fight.

Because nothing else seemed to work, I even tried bribing her with goodies and gifts. When you're desperate for rest, you'll do a lot of things to get it! It's not that I was a wimpy mother; it's that I was a worn-out woman.

Actually, to be honest, I can relate to my daughter because I fight my own body's cry for rest, especially if I think I am missing out on fun, food, or finishing my to-do list.

Soul Food

. . . .

God has told his people, "Here is a place of rest; let the weary rest here. This is a place of quiet rest." But they would not listen.

ISAIAH 28:12

I think there are a lot of reasons why we women struggle to be still and rest in our Lord. In our heads, we know rest is a gift from God; however, it is hard to rest when our spirits feel restless. There's always something to do, and if we haven't overcommitted ourselves, someone else needs us to get up from our place of rest and do something for him or her. We rarely allow ourselves to rest in the Lord and enjoy the gift of refreshment and relaxation.

Too many times we do not lay ourselves down until we are forced to by some sort of sickness. That's not God's plan. He wants us to rest our physical bodies, our minds, and our souls. This is not something we need to feel bad about—it does not mean we are weak. Quite the opposite, in fact: we can conquer more if we will take the time to allow the Lord to strengthen our bodies and our souls by embracing the blessing when we rest.

I invite you now to take a vacation from your problems and consider the New Life Recipes to help you get the rest and relaxation that you crave and deserve and that our Lord desires for you to have.

New Life Recipes

1. BATHE YOUR BODY AND SOUL

Purify me from my sins, and I will be clean;
wash me, and I will be whiter than snow.

PSALM 51:7

There is nothing sweeter for a woman than a quiet, warm, soothing bath. One of the most famous commercials targeted to women uses the slogan, "Calgon, take me away!" This tagline is for a bubble bath, and the manufacturer promises its product will give users rest and relaxation.

As good as the marketing is behind this commercial, nothing is more relaxing than resting in the Lord. If you're craving rest and relaxation, consider drawing a bath for yourself tonight. Put on some quiet worship music and let the Lord minister to you in that warm water. To get the full benefit, be sure to let your mind rest from your worries while you soak in the water and in worship!

2. TAKE A VACATION FROM YOUR WORRIES

Give all your worries and cares to God, for he cares about you.

I PETER 5:7

List all the things that make you restless so you can rest in the Lord. This, of course, is much easier said than done. Take a moment and write out a list of every burden you carry. Then take that list and hold it up toward heaven. Say these words out loud: "God, I give all of my worries to You, and in exchange I receive rest for my soul, mind, and body."

3. TREAT YOURSELF TO AN EARLY BEDTIME AND/OR A DAILY TWENTY-MINUTE NAP

God gives rest to his loved ones.

PSALM 127:2

If you're anything like me, once everything settles down in your home at night, you often get a burst of energy that drives you to try to get everything done into all hours of the night. Now I know there's no way you could convince me not to take advantage of those moments, and I suspect the same is true for you. If so, be sure to treat yourself to an early bedtime a few times a week. Write it on your calendar as if it were an appointment that can't be missed. If necessary, start with just one day. Once you do, you will begin to crave rest more than checking off another item on your out-of-control to-do lists.

POWER UP WITH PRAYER

God's promise of entering his rest still stands, so we ought to tremble with fear that some of you might fail to experience it.

HEBREWS 4:1

Dear God,
I want to receive Your gift of rest and experience the amazing refreshment that You offer when I rest my body and my spirit. Help me to let go of the little things and to embrace that rest again. Show me whatever I need to let go of so I can find refreshment and relaxation once again. Amen.

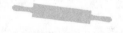

FOOD TRUTH

No food . . . is more delicious than the peace that comes from resting in the Lord.

Healthy Comfort Food Recipes

Now that we've talked about rest for our souls, let's make some healthy alternatives to the comfort foods that we all know and love, as well as foods that can help us relax from some of the stress life can create.

NOT-REALLY-CHEESE CHEESE SAUCE!

Serves 8

Ingredients:

2 cups raw macadamia nuts

2 cups cashews

Juice from 1 or 2 lemons (about ¼ cup)

1 clove garlic

½ tablespoon Butter Buds

Directions:

1. Place all ingredients in a blender and blend until the mixture is smooth. It will be thick! If it is too thick, you can add a little water.
2. Serve drizzled over meat, or use as a healthy cheese dip for nachos.

Recipe tip:

Go ahead and add more garlic or lemon to make it more flavorful. Get creative! Add chopped bell peppers to make it sweet, or if you like salty cheese, add sea salt. This will keep for three to five days in the fridge.

CAULI MAC 'N' CHEESE

Serves 4–6

Ingredients:

1 head cauliflower

2 cups whole-grain or gluten-free macaroni (elbow, bow tie, or
    twist noodles)

6 ounces Parmesan or Monterey Jack cheese, grated

1½ cups cheese sauce (use Not-Really-Cheese Cheese Sauce!; see
    page 19)

1 teaspoon sea salt

1 tablespoon onion powder

1 small bunch fresh parsley, chopped fine (optional)

Directions:

1. Slice off the stem of the cauliflower and cut or break head into
   small florets.
2. Cook pasta and cauliflower florets together in a large pot,
   according to the cooking directions for the pasta. Drain.
3. Mix Parmesan or Monterey Jack cheese with cheese sauce; add
   sea salt, onion powder, and parsley.
4. Mix pasta and cauliflower with cheese sauce and pour into
   serving bowl.

Recipe tip:

*Add chopped chicken to the mac 'n' cheese for some extra protein!
The mac 'n' cheese will keep in the fridge for two to three days.*

HEALTHY MAYONNAISE*

Makes about 2 cups

Ingredients:

½ cup water

½ cup macadamia nuts

¾ cup cashews

¼ teaspoon sea salt

1½ teaspoons apple cider vinegar

1 tablespoon freshly squeezed or bottled lemon juice

½ teaspoon Butter Buds

Directions:

1. Place all ingredients in a blender and blend until smooth.
2. Thin to desired consistency with water.

Recipe tip:

Use this recipe in tuna, egg, or potato salad—any recipe that calls for mayonnaise. Get creative with the flavor by adding different dried herbs or curry powder.

*Adapted from a recipe by Karen Knowler, The Raw Food Coach. See TheRawFoodCoach.com.

POTATO SALAD IN THE RAW

Serves 4–6

Ingredients:

5 large sweet potatoes, boiled and cooled

1 bunch green onions, sliced (about ½ cup)

1 handful chopped fresh chives

½ cup chopped red onion

½ cup thinly chopped red cabbage

¾ cup Healthy Mayonnaise (see recipe on page 21; use more or
   less to taste)

Directions:

1. Chop the sweet potatoes into bite-size pieces and place in
   a bowl.
2. Add green onions, chives, red onion, and red cabbage to the
   sweet potato pieces. Stir gently to mix.
3. Add Healthy Mayonnaise to potato mixture and stir gently
   to mix.

Recipe tip:

*This is a great entrée or a side dish to chicken. You can use
leftovers as a snack with whole-grain or gluten-free crackers
or other snack crackers for dipping.*

CORN CHOWDER
Serves 4–6

Ingredients:

6–8 ears corn or 2 cans (15 ounces each) whole kernel corn

4 cups skim or plain rice milk

2 tablespoons butter

1 teaspoon garlic powder

½ teaspoon sea salt

Freshly ground pepper

1 tablespoon minced fresh parsley (optional)

2 tablespoons honey

Directions:

1. If using fresh corn, cut kernels from the cobs into a large bowl. Then scrape the cobs with a spoon to extract the liquid.
2. Coat a large pot with nonstick spray and place over medium-low heat.
3. Add corn, milk, butter, garlic powder, sea salt, pepper (to taste), and parsley to the pan. Cook for about 10 minutes, stirring constantly.
4. When chowder is almost done, add the honey and stir well. Remove from heat and serve.

Recipe tip:

The starch in the corn will have a tendency to stick and burn easily, so be sure to stir the mixture regularly while the chowder is cooking.

HEALTHY CORN BREAD

Serves 10–12

Ingredients:

1 cup whole-grain or gluten-free flour

1 cup cornmeal

¼ cup raw sugar

1 teaspoon baking soda

¾ teaspoon salt

1 cup plain nonfat yogurt

2 eggs, beaten

Directions:

1. Preheat oven to 400° and lightly grease an 8 x 8-inch baking pan.
2. Mix flour, cornmeal, sugar, baking soda, and salt in a large bowl. Add the yogurt and eggs. Stir until well blended.
3. Pour batter into prepared pan and bake for 20 to 25 minutes, or until the center of the corn bread is springy when pressed.

Recipe tip:

Enjoy this delicious corn bread with your favorite chili or the Corn Chowder recipe on page 23.

SOFT-SERVE CHAMOMILE VANILLA ICE CREAM

Serves 1–2

Ingredients:

1 cup of hot water

4 chamomile tea bags

2 cans (16 ounces each) coconut milk or 4 cups rice milk

1 teaspoon vanilla extract

1 cup honey

2 cups ice

Directions:

1. Steep tea in hot water; let cool. Make the tea about 30 minutes before you want to eat the ice cream so that it has time to cool in the fridge.
2. Put all ingredients in a blender and mix. For soft-serve, scoop into small serving dishes and enjoy. For firmer ice cream, put in freezer at least 1½ hours before serving.

Recipe tip:

Make brownies to go along with this recipe of soft-serve ice cream, loaded with the benefits of chamomile.

TASTE OF TRUTH

Rest is a gift to you from God Himself.

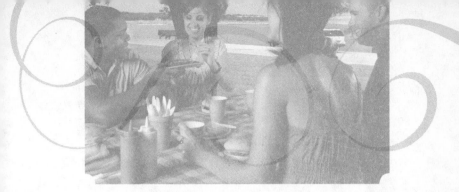

CHAPTER 3

Craving Something Different

*Weird, Wonderful Recipes and
Becoming a Bizarre Blessing*

I WAS RAISED with a very weird and wonderful father. In fact, if you often crave something different, you would have liked having my father as your best friend!

On one of my stepmother's birthdays, my dad decided to give her a different kind of birthday gift. She loved elephants; she collected and displayed them all over our home. So my wacky father decided to have Marine World/Africa USA deliver a live elephant to the door of our home!

My dad didn't stop there. He had contacted three different news stations to cover the story. Their camera crews filmed animal trainers helping my mom up on the saddle of the elephant and then parading her around our neighborhood. Although our neighbors were afraid to come out and watch, you could see their startled faces looking out the windows of every house in our cul-de-sac.

Soul Food
. . . .

God works in different ways, but it is the same God who does the work in all of us.

1 CORINTHIANS 12:6

From the day that elephant paid his house call, our neighbors never again invited us to their home for barbecues. They were somewhat distant though always pleasant—probably out of fear of what might be delivered to their door!

Sometimes I think we respond just like those neighbors. We put God in a box and forget the very different and divine ways our Lord delivers blessings to us. Rarely does He display His power or direct our lives in an ordinary way.

Think about the bizarre way He blessed many of His chosen ones in the Bible. He blessed David in front of a giant; He blessed Daniel by rescuing him from a lions' den; He blessed Moses in front of what appeared to be a sea of hopelessness but actually became the grand entrance to the Promised Land.

Too many times we crave something different from what God has planned for us, thinking it will bring us an adventure. What we're really craving, though, is a purpose-driven life filled with God adventures. Believe me, if we're prayed up, purposed, and prepared, we will find exactly what we're looking for!

When we're bored with our faith and craving something different, I believe it is because God does not want us to settle for less than what He has for us.

Deep down in the heart of every person there is a craving to make a difference, to do something that sets him or her apart. That is a God-given desire, and He has designed each of us for a very different purpose. We do not have to aspire to become Christian clones or live out our faith walk like our friends do. Yes, we learn from one another, but we are not supposed to become anything other than who God made us to be.

If you are looking for a different and divine God experience that will give you a better and bigger picture of how our weird and wonderful God works differently in each of our lives, see the following New Life Recipes.

New Life Recipes

1. WATCH *IT'S A WONDERFUL LIFE*

Such knowledge is too wonderful for me,
too great for me to understand!

PSALM 139:6

This holiday classic stars Jimmy Stewart as George Bailey, a small-town banker who is never able to escape his hometown and fulfill his dream of world travel. The movie didn't do much at the box office when it was first released in 1946. Only when its copyright expired in the 1970s, making it an inexpensive program for TV stations to air, did a large number of viewers come to cherish the story of how an angel named Clarence showed the despairing George how significant his life really was.

I realize this movie is usually watched at Christmastime. However, it gives such a clear picture of how we can overlook unseen blessings that I recommend you watch it anytime you wonder whether God is really using you. You'll also be reminded how wonderful your life really is when it's lived for the greater cause of helping others.

2. LOOK AHEAD EXPECTANTLY

I heard a loud shout from the throne, saying, "Look, God's home is now among his people! He will live with them, and they will be his people. God himself will be with them. He will wipe every tear from their eyes,

*and there will be no more death or sorrow or crying or pain. All these
things are gone forever."*

*And the one sitting on the throne said, "Look, I am making everything
new!" And then he said to me, "Write this down, for what I tell you is
trustworthy and true."*

REVELATION 21:3-5

When you fight to find a blessing, remember and meditate on these
trustworthy words above.

3. BECOME A BIZARRE BLESSING

*Abigail wasted no time. She quickly gathered 200 loaves of bread, two
wineskins full of wine, five sheep that had been slaughtered, nearly a
bushel of roasted grain, 100 clusters of raisins, and 200 fig cakes. She
packed them on donkeys.*

I SAMUEL 25:18

Abigail was a bizarre blessing, and she was blessed because of it. Her
husband, Nabal, made David mad by refusing to feed David's army
after David and his men had protected Nabal's flocks in the wilderness.
As David was on his way to kill her husband, Abigail met him and,
with wise and humble words, persuaded David not to harm Nabal. As
a result, David changed his mind and praised God for Abigail's good
sense, which had kept him from shedding blood. Not long after, when
her foolish husband died, David even took Abigail as his wife!

POWER UP WITH PRAYER

*You made all the delicate, inner parts of my body and knit me together in
my mother's womb. Thank you for making me so wonderfully complex!
Your workmanship is marvelous—how well I know it. You watched me
as I was being formed in utter seclusion, as I was woven together in the
dark of the womb. You saw me before I was born. Every day of my life was*

recorded in your book. Every moment was laid out before a single day had passed. How precious are your thoughts about me, O God. They cannot be numbered!

PSALM 139:13-17

Heavenly Father,
Sometimes I struggle to see myself as wonderfully complex.
I'm humbled when I realize how much You value me. Help
me to begin seeing myself—and everyone I meet—as one
of Your unique and irreplaceable creatures. In Jesus' name,
amen.

FOOD TRUTH

No food . . . will ever fill us up more than doing God's will.

Weird and Wonderful Food Recipes

Are you tired of eating the same foods and feeling unhealthy? It's time for a recipe makeover! Here are some incredible recipes that are unique and delicious.

GLAZED GREEN BEANS AND YAMS

Serves 6

Ingredients:

1 cup plus 3 tablespoons water

3 large yams

1 pound fresh green beans

1½ teaspoons butter

1 tablespoon freshly squeezed or bottled lemon juice

1 teaspoon gluten-free or whole-grain flour

1 teaspoon grated lemon peel

2 tablespoons chopped nuts (such as almonds, pecans, or cashews)

Directions:

1. Slice yams diagonally about ¼-inch thick. This should make about 2 cups.
2. Place 1 cup water in a 10-inch skillet and bring to a boil.
3. Reduce to medium heat. Add green beans and yams to skillet. Cover and cook 5 to 8 minutes until the green beans and yams are crisp-tender, stirring occasionally. Drain and remove from skillet; keep warm.
4. Melt butter in the same skillet.
5. In a small bowl, stir together lemon juice, flour, and 3 tablespoons water. Add to the melted butter. Cook over medium heat, stirring occasionally until sauce thickens, about 2 to 3 minutes.
6. Stir in the lemon peel just before removing from heat.
7. To serve, spoon sauce over green beans and yams. Sprinkle the chopped nuts on top.

CARROT AND ALMOND DIP

Makes about 2 cups; serves 4

Ingredients:

2 cups almonds

2 large carrots

½ cup coarsely chopped red onion

½ cup finely chopped fresh parsley

¼ cup freshly squeezed or bottled lemon juice

1 pinch sea salt

1 teaspoon garlic powder

Directions:

1. Soak almonds in a bowl of water overnight.
2. Boil carrots until soft.
3. Combine softened carrots, almonds, and the rest of the ingredients in a blender. Mix until smooth.
4. Add water for desired consistency.
5. Serve as a dip for veggies or crackers.

Recipe tip:

You don't have to use almonds—try walnuts or even cashews instead. This recipe can also be used as a sauce for meat.

THAT'S A WRAP!

Serves 4

Ingredients for wraps:

8 white cabbage leaves

2 avocados, sliced

2 tomatoes, diced

1 cup black olives, sliced

¼ cup chopped cilantro

1 medium zucchini, grated

Ingredients for dip:

¼ cup olive oil

1 tablespoon freshly squeezed or bottled lemon juice

¼ cup chopped cilantro

1 tablespoon finely chopped fresh ginger

¼ cup pressed garlic

¼ cup water (optional)

1 teaspoon onion powder

Directions for wraps:

1. Lay open the cabbage leaves. Divide vegetables equally among cabbage leaves, placing avocado slices and tomato in the middle of each leaf, then adding black olives, 1½ teaspoons cilantro, and zucchini for each serving.
2. Fold cabbage leaves up into wraps.

Directions for dip:

1. Pour olive oil into a small bowl. Add lemon juice and cilantro.
2. Mix the ginger with the garlic.
3. Combine olive oil mixture with the ginger and garlic, adding water if the mixture seems too oily. Mix in onion powder.
4. Use as a dipping sauce for the wraps.

Recipe tip:

The dipping sauce is also good as a salad dressing or vegetable dip.

SPINACH CREAM SOUP

Serves 2–3

Ingredients:

2 teaspoons olive oil

2 cups portobello mushrooms

1 bag spinach

3 cups water

1 can (16 ounces) coconut milk

2 tablespoons dried minced onion

2 tablespoons butter

3 tablespoons chicken bouillon powder

Directions:

1. Warm oil in a skillet over medium heat. Add mushrooms and cook until mushrooms are softened.
2. Combine spinach and softened mushrooms in a blender until smooth. Set aside.
3. Bring water to a boil in a large saucepan. Add coconut milk, onion, butter, and bouillon.
4. Add spinach and mushroom puree to the mixture in saucepan; stir and cook on medium heat for 5 to 7 minutes or until soup thickens, stirring occasionally.

Recipe tip:

Don't be afraid to experiment—sprinkle shredded Parmesan cheese on soup or get creative with spices to change the flavor.

GRILLED PORTOBELLO MUSHROOM BURGERS

Serves 4

Ingredients:

4 portobello mushroom caps

1 tablespoon minced garlic

¼ teaspoon sea salt

2 tablespoons olive oil

1 onion, sliced

4 whole-grain buns

1 tomato, sliced

4 lettuce leaves

¼ cup low-fat or Healthy Mayonnaise (see page 21), or to taste

¼ teaspoon low-sodium soy sauce or Bragg Liquid Aminos

Directions:

1. Place mushroom caps, smooth side up, in a shallow dish. In a small bowl, mix garlic and sea salt to taste. Pour over the mushrooms. Let sit at room temperature for 15 minutes.
2. Preheat grill to medium-high heat.
3. Brush grate with 1½ tablespoons oil. Place mushrooms on the grill for 5 to 8 minutes on each side, or until tender.
4. Meanwhile, sauté onion slices in 2 teaspoons olive oil in a skillet until tender.
5. Toast whole-grain buns.
6. Add cooked mushrooms to bottom halves of buns and top with tomato, onion slices, and lettuce. Mix desired amount of mayonnaise with soy sauce or Bragg Liquid Aminos. Pour mayonnaise mixture onto mushroom burgers and cover with tops of buns. Enjoy!

ZUCCHINI PANCAKES

Serves 2–3

Ingredients:

4 medium zucchini, shredded and drained

3 medium red onions, chopped

1 clove garlic, minced

2 eggs, slightly beaten

½ teaspoon sea salt

1 pinch pepper

⅓ cup crumbled feta or farmer cheese

2 tablespoons whole-grain or gluten-free flour

½ teaspoon oregano

½ teaspoon basil

Directions:

1. Combine all ingredients and mix well.
2. Coat a nonstick skillet with cooking spray and place over medium-high heat.
3. Drop zucchini mixture one tablespoonful at a time onto the skillet to make small pancakes. Cook about one minute, then turn pancakes over to brown the other side for one more minute. Serve immediately or freeze for later.

Recipe tip:

To cook as a casserole, pour the mixture into a greased 9 x 13-inch pan and bake at 350° for 20 minutes. Cut and serve.

SQUASH STIR-FRY

Serves 4–6

Ingredients:

2 medium zucchini, sliced

2 medium crookneck (yellow) squash, sliced

½ cup red bell pepper, julienned

¼ cup diced red onion

¼ teaspoon basil

¼ teaspoon oregano

1 teaspoon butter

1 clove garlic, minced

Sea salt

Freshly ground pepper

Directions:

1. Coat a skillet with nonstick spray and place over medium-high heat.
2. Place zucchini, squash, red bell pepper, and onion in the pan and sauté for 3 to 5 minutes.
3. Add herbs and butter, stirring for 2 to 3 minutes more.
4. Add garlic. Turn off heat and blend well. Season to taste with salt and pepper, if desired, and enjoy.

Recipe tip:

Add diced cooked chicken breast to this recipe, and you have an easy, low-fat entrée. Yum!

TASTE OF TRUTH

**You were not created to fit in;
you are divinely different
to stand out.**

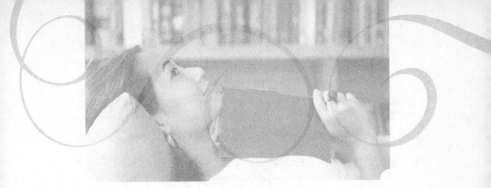

CHAPTER 4

Craving Zest for Life

Salty, Satisfying Recipes and
Faith Seasonings for Life's Seasons

SEVERAL YEARS AGO while I was on a book tour, I had a craving for something salty. Unfortunately, my craving was out of control, and I ate an extra-large bag of potato chips all by myself while watching a movie.

The next day I had a television interview about a book I had just written on health. I don't eat salt very often, and when I woke up that morning, my eyes were swollen shut from the high sodium intake the night before. No amount of ice or Preparation H cream underneath my eyes could bring the swelling down. To this day, I dread seeing that interview, which is posted on YouTube. I looked as if I had been punched in both eyes. The good news, though, is that God can work even through puffy eyes and thighs!

Soul Food
· ·

*Salt is good for seasoning. But if it loses its flavor, how do you make it salty
again? You must have the qualities of salt among yourselves and live in
peace with each other.*

MARK 9:50

Many of us have moments of weakness when we feel as if our cravings
have taken us captive or left us out of control. Sometimes they leave our
faith flavorless because we are craving what used to be or what we wish
could be. The Bible tells us there is a season for everything, and if we
don't learn to taste each season as it is served, we will end up missing
special moments and those life lessons we need to draw closer to God.

I love the seasons of love and laughter, but I have discovered that the
seasons of loneliness and painful places are when I learn what my faith
is for. The best way to season our faith again is to become salt in others'
lives when our own feels lifeless. I offer a few other ideas in the following
New Life Recipes.

New Life Recipes
· ·

1. TRY A NEW FLAVOR

Taste and see that the LORD is good.
    Oh, the joys of those who take refuge in him!
PSALM 34:8

If you are craving more flavor in your faith walk, pick up a new Christian
book to read or find a new Christian friend to hang out with.

If your church does not help you grow closer to God, don't be afraid
to try a new church. The great thing about all the different ways and
styles of Christian churches is that you and I have the freedom to look

for the one that stimulates our faith and works best with our gifts and personality.

2. SING A NEW SONG

Sing a new song to the LORD! Let the whole earth sing to the LORD!
    PSALM 96:1

Worship should bring joy and flavor to our faith. Find some new worship songs that fit the style of music you love to listen to. If you're craving closeness with God, sing a new song, or better yet, sit down and write a song to the Lord, putting it to your own melody.

3. PURIFY YOURSELF

Then he went out to the spring that supplied the town with water and threw the salt into it. And he said, "This is what the LORD says: I have purified this water. It will no longer cause death or infertility."
    2 KINGS 2:21

Many times we can't taste God's goodness because we have been feeding our soul salt substitutes instead of real faith. In other words, we watch, read, and listen to things that go against everything we want to become in Christ. We lose our craving for the Word and attempt to satisfy our soul with unhealthy, man-made forms of entertainment. Just like a whole-food diet makes us crave healthier foods, a pure soul-food cleanse will get rid of the junk in our spirits so we can taste God's goodness again.

POWER UP WITH PRAYER

Let your good deeds shine out for all to see, so that everyone will praise your heavenly Father.
    MATTHEW 5:16

Dear God,
I pray that You will increase my craving for You and fill
me up so full that salt and goodness will spill out onto
those I love. Show me the artificial things in my life that
are keeping me from tasting and becoming Your salt to this
world. Amen.

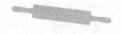

FOOD TRUTH
No food . . . is as savory as God's favor, strength, and wisdom.

Salty and Satisfying Food Recipes

We all know salty foods aren't necessarily the best for us, so why do we crave salt so much? Instead of having a salty main dish, we should be eating healthier entrées with salty foods on the side. Here are some great recipes that are sure to satisfy your salty craving without sending your health overboard.

OUI OUI ONION SOUP

Serves 4

Ingredients:

1 tablespoon butter

1 tablespoon olive oil

3 large onions

¼ teaspoon sea salt

1 teaspoon raw sugar

1 tablespoon whole-grain or gluten-free flour

⅓ cup dry cooking sherry

6 cups reduced-sodium chicken broth

¼ teaspoon freshly ground black pepper

2 teaspoons low-sodium soy sauce or Bragg Liquid Aminos

Directions:

1. In a heavy skillet, heat butter and olive oil. Add onions and salt. Cook 5 minutes, covered, then uncover and add sugar.
2. Cook, stirring frequently for 15 to 25 minutes or until onions are golden brown.
3. Add flour and reduce heat to medium. Cook for 1 minute.
4. Add sherry, scraping skillet frequently. Cook 1 to 2 minutes or until slightly reduced.
5. Transfer to a saucepan. Add broth and pepper and bring to a boil.
6. Reduce heat to low and simmer, covered, for 10 minutes. Add soy sauce or Bragg Liquid Aminos.

MOTO STACK
Serves 2–4

Ingredients:

4 ounces fresh mozzarella roll, sliced

3 large ripe tomatoes, sliced into ¼-inch slices

10 basil leaves (optional)

3 tablespoons balsamic vinegar

2 teaspoons sea salt

Directions:

1. Place a mozzarella slice on top of each tomato slice, and then place a basil leaf on top of the mozzarella.
2. Arrange stacks on a plate, drizzle balsamic vinegar evenly over each stack, sprinkle with salt, and enjoy!

Recipe tip:

This can also be turned into a great salad—slice cherry tomatoes in half, cut smaller mozzarella pieces, add spinach and basil leaves (if desired); use balsamic vinegar as the dressing. It is simply divine!

MOUTHWATERING MELON BITES

Serves 2–3

Ingredients:

2 cups sliced cantaloupe

14 slices prosciutto

Directions:

1. Wrap slices of prosciutto around individual pieces of cantaloupe.
2. Hold together with toothpicks. Serve and enjoy!

Recipe tip:

This recipe is so simple and delicious—a great finger food for a party. Try switching out the melon for kalamata olives. Yum!

QUESO FIESTA DIP

Serves 3–4

Ingredients:

1 small onion, chopped

1 teaspoon olive oil

2 garlic cloves, minced

1 package (8 ounces) low-fat cream cheese, cubed

2 cups fresh diced tomatoes

6 ounces shredded cheddar cheese

1 teaspoon chili powder

½ pound lean ground beef, cooked

1 can (8 ounces) green chilies

1 bag tortilla chips

Directions:

1. In a large skillet, sauté onion in oil until tender. Add garlic and cream cheese and stir until cream cheese is melted. Add tomatoes, cheddar cheese, chili powder, ground beef, and green chilies. Mix thoroughly.
2. Stir over low heat until cheddar cheese is melted.
3. Keep warm; serve with tortilla chips.

Recipe tip:

Add cilantro for more flavor and jalapeños for more spice!

WRAP ME UP!

Serves 1

Ingredients:

1 whole-grain tortilla

1 Laughing Cow cheese wedge, original flavor

3 or 4 lettuce leaves

3 slices smoked turkey

2 slices cooked turkey bacon

Directions:

1. Spread cheese evenly on tortilla.
2. Place lettuce, turkey, and bacon on tortilla.
3. Roll up and enjoy!

Recipe tip:

Add slices of tomato and/or olives for more saltiness.

KALE CHIPS

Serves 2–3

Ingredients:

1 head kale, washed and dried

1 teaspoon olive oil

1 teaspoon salt

Directions:

1. Preheat oven to 350°.
2. Line a baking sheet with parchment paper.
3. Remove stems from kale; chop leaves into one-inch pieces.
4. Combine all ingredients in a bowl and mix with your hands.
5. Spread kale in a single layer on prepared baking sheet.
6. Bake for 10 to 13 minutes, until dry and crispy. Cool for 10 minutes and serve.

Recipe tip:

Try using eggplant instead of, or along with, the kale. Slice the eggplant thin and prepare it the same way as the kale.

PEANUT BUTTER PICKLE DELIGHT

Serves 2–4

Ingredients:

2 whole dill pickles

3 tablespoons peanut butter

2 rice cakes

Directions:

1. Slice the pickles into rounds, about six to an inch.
2. Spread peanut butter on rice cakes.
3. Place pickle slices side by side on top of the peanut butter and enjoy!

Recipe tip:

This is seriously delicious. If you are allergic to peanuts, try using almond or cashew butter instead.

TASTE OF TRUTH

**Life will lose its flavor if it is not
seasoned with faith, hope, and love.**

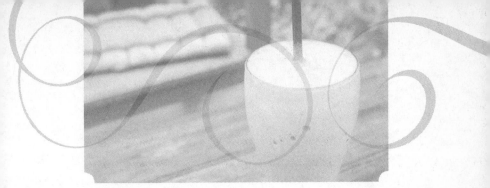

CHAPTER 5

Craving God's Sweet Presence

Real Sweet Recipes and Some Sweet Jesus Time

YEARS AGO when my husband and I were first married, we made a commitment to fast from sugar for thirty days. I have to be honest—it was the hardest thing I'd ever done, and I didn't make it. Steve was craving a breakthrough from God and fasting for the right reasons. I, on the other hand, was not fasting to draw closer to God but to impress my new husband. I was miserable without my treats.

Then I remembered that there was a frozen wedding cake in my freezer and sharp knives (wedding gifts) in my kitchen drawers. Each day when Steve would leave for work, I would grab a knife and open the freezer; then I would take out the frozen wedding cake, tip it upside down, and carve out a piece from the center. It was heavenly—until I got caught. A few weeks after I'd started my nibbling, my husband opened up the freezer and something fell onto the foiled wedding cake. With nothing left but a fragile shell of icing, it crumbled. I had eaten every ounce of cake in the center.

Soul Food

. . . .

> *My child, eat honey, for it is good,*
>   *and the honeycomb is sweet to the taste.*
>
> PROVERBS 24:13

I don't think there's anything wrong with eating something sweet, but I now know there is nothing better than the sweet presence of our Lord and Savior and eating the food He created for our bodies and taste buds to enjoy.

The good news is we do not have to fight our craving for sweets anymore; we just need to treat ourselves to God's goodness of natural sweeteners like honey, molasses, pure maple syrup, and stevia. I can't think of anything more satisfying than good, healthy sweets and sweet time with our Lord.

Today many health professionals advocate cutting back or eliminating white sugar from our diets altogether. If you choose to take this step, don't think of white sugar as something you have to give up; think of it as something you get to give up so you can experience sweet health benefits and the adventure of finding healthy treats to eat. Here are some sweet ideas to satisfy your soul as you discover new ways to taste and see that the Lord is good!

New Life Recipes

. . . .

1. SING SWEET LOVE SONGS TO JESUS

> *Sing praises to God, sing praises;*
>   *sing praises to our King, sing praises!*
>
> PSALM 47:6

Love songs captivate our hearts but leave us longing for love from a man that we may never find. Let's try to sing those same love songs to the one true Prince who will always give us what we are really craving. Take a moment to play your favorite love song and sing it to the Lord. You may have to alter the words a bit, but if your heart is fixed on connecting to Jesus, the words will overflow from your mouth and your heart will feel His sweet presence.

2. EAT SWEETS AND READ THE WORD

How sweet your words taste to me;
they are sweeter than honey.

PSALM 119:103

If you struggle with being still and spending sweet time with Jesus, then try making a healthy treat like some of the ones in this chapter. Then sit and dine with your Lord. Just as we eat popcorn and candy while watching a two-hour movie—can you imagine if a healthy snack helped you sit and savor time with your Lord? Now that would be a treat!

3. WRITE NOTES TO JESUS

And you must love the LORD your God with all your heart, all your soul,
all your mind, and all your strength.

MARK 12:30

Keep Post-it notes by your bed, and whenever you have a craving to express love to someone, turn that love toward heaven. Write love notes to Jesus and post them on your mirror as a reminder of the love relationship you are developing with your Savior.

POWER UP WITH PRAYER

The commandments of the LORD are right,
bringing joy to the heart. . . .
They are more desirable than gold,

even the finest gold.
They are sweeter than honey,
    even honey dripping from the comb.
PSALM 19:8, 10

Dear Jesus,
Your commandments are right; let them bring joy to my
heart. I want Your commands to make me wise, giving me
insight for pure living and everlasting reverence. You are
more desirable than gold, even the finest gold. Your Word
is sweeter than honey, even honey dripping from the comb.
Amen.

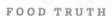

FOOD TRUTH

No food . . . tastes as sweet as a fruitful day.

"Real" Sweet Guilt-Free Recipes

I love sweets and crave them often. I can't imagine life without sweet treats! In fact, I always seem to somehow find a way to alter every sweet-tasting recipe into a healthy version. Here are some of my favorites.

BROWN RICE CUSTARD

Serves 2–4

Ingredients:

3 eggs, lightly beaten

1 teaspoon pure vanilla extract

½ cup rice, almond, or coconut milk

1 teaspoon cinnamon

½ teaspoon nutmeg

¼ teaspoon sea salt

¼ cup honey

2 cups cooked brown rice

Directions:

1. Preheat oven to 325°.
2. Combine eggs, vanilla, milk, cinnamon, nutmeg, sea salt, and honey. Mix well.
3. Stir in cooked rice.
4. Pour the mixture into a 9 x 13-inch nonstick baking pan.
5. Bake 35 to 40 minutes, or until a toothpick inserted into the center comes out clean.
6. Cool to room temperature. Scoop into dessert dishes or cut into squares.

Recipe tip:

You could add raisins or dried cranberries to this recipe. Get creative and add your favorite fruit!

RASPBERRY PEACH SMOOTHIE

Serves 1

Ingredients:

½ cup warm raspberry tea, brewed strong

3 tablespoons honey

1 cup peaches, diced

½ cup raspberries

¾ cup low-fat, plain organic yogurt

6 ice cubes

Directions:

1. Dissolve honey in warm tea. Refrigerate until chilled.
2. Combine the sweetened tea, peaches, raspberries, yogurt, and ice in a blender and mix until smooth.

Recipe tip:

This could be an incredible breakfast. You can also experiment with other fruits instead of peaches—think mangoes with raspberries!

SWEET MINT PIE*

Serves 12

Ingredients for crust:

2 cups ground almonds

½ cup unsweetened dark cocoa powder

¼ cup agave syrup or raw honey

2 tablespoons coconut or grapeseed oil

¼ cup semisweet chocolate chips

1 pinch sea salt

Directions for crust:

1. Pulse all ingredients together in a blender.
2. Pour into a standard 9-inch pie pan. Press with your fingers to form the pie crust.

Ingredients for mint filling:

1 cup water

1 cup agave syrup or honey

1 teaspoon mint extract

1 tablespoon butter

1 tablespoon raw sugar or agave syrup

1½ cups cashew butter

Directions for mint filling:

1. Place all ingredients in a blender and blend until smooth.
2. Pour filling into the crust.

Ingredients for pie topping:

1½ cups butter

½ cup semisweet chocolate chips

1 cup unsweetened dark cocoa powder

¼ cup agave syrup or honey

1 tablespoon coconut or grapeseed oil

¼ teaspoon peppermint extract

Directions for pie topping:

1. Melt butter.
2. Melt chocolate chips in a double boiler or in a small saucepan placed in a larger pan containing boiling water.
3. Mix with remaining ingredients.
4. Pour evenly over mint filling.
5. Keep in freezer at least one hour until ready to serve.

Recipe tip:

This is great for parties or when you're craving a refreshing treat. The mint is oh so tasty!

*Adapted from Nina Dench's recipe for Karen Knowler, The Raw Food Coach. See TheRawFoodCoach.com.

HEAVENLY APPLES AND BANANAS
Serves 4–6

Ingredients:

6 very ripe bananas, sliced

4 apples, sliced thin

1 teaspoon cinnamon

½ teaspoon nutmeg

1 teaspoon vanilla extract

1 tablespoon raw sugar or stevia

Directions:

1. Coat a skillet with nonstick spray and place over medium-high heat.
2. Place bananas in skillet and stir until they begin to brown.
3. Add apples to bananas and mix. Sauté until the apples are tender when pierced with a fork.
4. Stir in cinnamon, nutmeg, and vanilla at the last minute of sautéing.
5. Turn off heat. Evenly sprinkle the raw sugar or stevia over the fruit. Spoon into dessert dishes and serve.

Recipe tip:

Add a scoop of your favorite vanilla ice cream and you will have a spoonful of heaven! You can serve this dish warm or cold.

BANANA BLISS PIE*

Serves 8–10

Ingredients for crust:

3 cups oatmeal, blended to a fine powder

1 cup crushed almonds

¾ cup honey

1 tablespoon almond or peanut butter

1 pinch sea salt

3 bananas

Directions for crust:

1. Preheat oven to 350°.
2. Mix all ingredients except bananas in a large bowl.
3. Place mixture in bottom of pie dish and pat down to form a crust, using your hands or a spatula.
4. Bake for 5 to 8 minutes, until the mixture seems firm.
5. Let cool for 5 minutes. Meanwhile, cut bananas into thin slices. When crust is cool, spread banana slices to cover the bottom pie crust.

Ingredients for toffee:

1 cup almond or peanut butter

1 cup maple syrup

1 pinch sea salt

Directions for toffee:

1. Mix all ingredients together until smooth.
2. Pour over bananas in crust.

Ingredients for pie topping:

5 bananas

1 cup almond or peanut butter

½ cup honey

½ teaspoon vanilla extract

Directions for pie topping:

1. Blend all ingredients until smooth and pour over toffee.
2. Place in fridge for an hour before serving.

*Adapted from Nina Dench's recipe for Karen Knowler, The Raw Food Coach. See TheRawFoodCoach.com.

BASIC VANILLA SHAKE

Serves 2

Ingredients:

2 cups vanilla Rice Dream ice cream or whole vanilla bean ice
    cream

1 teaspoon vanilla extract

1 tablespoon honey

1 cup ice (more if needed)

Directions:

1. Place all ingredients in blender.
2. Mix for 1 to 2 minutes, or until smooth. Pour and enjoy!

Recipe tip:

*Add a scoop of vanilla protein powder or oat bran to sneak
in some protein!*

CHAI YUM

Serves 1

Ingredients:

1 bag chai tea

1 packet stevia

1 dash coconut creamer

Directions:

Place chai tea bag in mug filled with hot water. Add stevia and creamer.

TASTE OF TRUTH

**Nothing sweet tastes better
than the Lord's presence, which
satisfies the soul.**

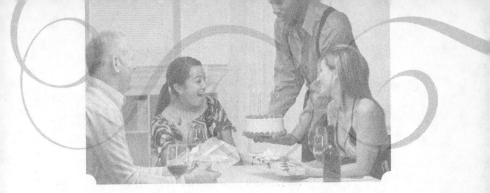

CHAPTER 6

Craving Life's Celebrations

Healthy Holiday Recipes and Happy Home Memories

"OPEN HAPPINESS."

This slogan, used by the Coca-Cola Company, is one that I love—and I don't even drink Coke! Much of this slogan's appeal, I believe, stems from our desire to experience happiness.

I think one reason we don't celebrate as much as we could is because we don't believe there's anything to celebrate. In fact, the longer we live, the more we realize how hard life can be. We have to fight to find joy.

I come from a broken home, so holidays could be a painful time for me if I allowed them to be. It seems that every year I am forced to make a choice between celebrating the present or looking back on the people I lost when my parents divorced. To be honest, it is always a battle, but I have found that if I cry out to God when I'm hurting and ask Him to help me embrace those He has placed in front of me, I always find something or someone to celebrate.

Soul Food
. . . .

There is nothing better than to be happy and enjoy ourselves as long as we can.

ECCLESIASTES 3:12

Notice that the wisest king who ever lived reminds you and me that good food and good friends are meant to be enjoyed throughout our lives. Don't feel guilty for craving happiness; instead, learn how to find your joy and happiness in things that are holy, everlasting, and worth celebrating. When you read through the Bible, you see that after every trial or battle won, there was a feast and celebration.

The battles in your life are not meant to keep you down; they are meant to keep you close to God and give you a way to find joy in spite of any circumstances, knowing that your God is faithful and will fight for you. In the following New Life Recipes I have listed three ideas that I believe will help you find the happiness you're craving and new ways to celebrate!

New Life Recipes
. . . .

1. LOOK FOR SOMETHING TO CELEBRATE

Fix your thoughts on what is true, and honorable, and right, and pure, and lovely, and admirable. Think about things that are excellent and worthy of praise.

PHILIPPIANS 4:8

I grew up in a home that was filled with fighting, and to be honest, nothing seemed worthy of celebration. I hear from many women who describe a similar environment in their own homes. They are discouraged by the conflict that drives out any sense of peace and well-being.

I know that when life is out of control, we tend to be blind to the many blessings that come each day. Take a moment and write out one thing worthy of praise. You can even start with the little things, like a sunny day, a flower, or food to eat. Then you can build the list from there.

2. SPEAK OF HEAVEN OFTEN

God himself will be with them. He will wipe every tear from their eyes, and there will be no more death or sorrow or crying or pain. All these things are gone forever.

REVELATION 21:3-4

In those seasons when it seems there is nothing to celebrate, you may need to look beyond the here and now to the bigger picture. At such times, allow your heart and mind to meditate on the things of heaven. Keep in mind that we're only here for a little while, and if you're in a season in which it seems there is nothing to celebrate, remember that we will be forever celebrating in heaven. Let your mind dwell on those things.

Read the Scripture above and let your heart celebrate the day when there will be no more sickness, no more death, and no more tears. Allow yourself to breathe in His presence and dream about the Savior's return. When you do, you will find a reason to celebrate.

3. CREATE CELEBRATIONS

In Jerusalem, the LORD of Heaven's Armies will spread a wonderful feast for all the people of the world. It will be a delicious banquet with clear, well-aged wine and choice meat.

ISAIAH 25:6

Feasting is very much a part of creating celebrations, and you can bring this joyful mood into your home every day. Decorate your table with fresh-cut flowers or set out your pretty dishes for no reason other than to say "I love you" to those in your household. Just before you eat, turn on some soft, beautiful instrumental music. Then light a candle and seal the attitude of celebration in your home with a prayer, asking for the joy of God's presence to fill your home.

POWER UP WITH PRAYER

Let them praise the LORD for his great love and for the wonderful things he has done for them. For he satisfies the thirsty and fills the hungry with good things.

PSALM 107:8-9

Help me, Lord, to praise You for Your great love and for the wonderful things You have done for me. Open my heart that I will be satisfied by You alone. May I thirst for You and be fulfilled with the good things You offer, now and forever. Amen.

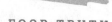

FOOD TRUTH

No food . . . is more delightful than celebrating a victory.

Craving a Happy Holiday: Healthy Holiday Recipes and Holy Ways to Host Holidays

Perhaps your cherished holiday memories include scenes of your family around the table enjoying the same dishes lovingly prepared and served year after year. Fortunately, you can make healthy versions of many of these foods without sacrificing great taste. Enjoy some of the following recipes at your next holiday meal—or anytime!

CAULI-MASHERS

Serves 6

Ingredients:

1 head cauliflower

1 tablespoon cream cheese

2 pressed garlic cloves

1 teaspoon fresh rosemary

1 teaspoon onion powder

¼ cup grated Parmesan cheese

¼ cup butter

⅛ teaspoon chicken bouillon powder

1 teaspoon sea salt, or to taste

⅛ teaspoon pepper, or to taste

Directions:

1. Bring a medium pot of water to boil and cut cauliflower into small pieces. Boil until tender and drain.
2. Using a hand mixer, mash the cauliflower with the cream cheese, garlic, rosemary, onion powder, Parmesan, butter, and bouillon.
3. Once all ingredients are mashed and mixed together, add sea salt and pepper.
4. Serve and enjoy!

Recipe tip:

This is an incredible substitute dish for mashed potatoes at Thanksgiving dinner.

HOMEMADE CRANBERRY SAUCE

Fills a medium-size bowl

Ingredients:

1 small (12 ounces) bag fresh or frozen cranberries

1 can (16 ounces) pineapple chunks in juice, undrained (if using fresh pineapple, about 2 cups)

1½ teaspoons orange zest

½ cup honey, stevia, or raw sugar

Directions:

1. Place cranberries, pineapple, pineapple juice, orange zest, and sweetener in food processor. Mix until all cranberries have been crushed.
2. If you'd like it sweeter, add one or two packets of stevia.
3. Pour mixture into bowl. Cover and chill until mealtime.

Recipe tip:

Add walnuts or pine nuts as a garnish right before serving.

STUFFED RED BELL PEPPER POPS

Serves 4–6

Ingredients:

4 red bell peppers

1 pound ground beef or turkey

½ teaspoon chopped garlic

½ cup chopped onion

2 teaspoons cumin

1 can (8 ounces) tomato sauce

1 cup cooked brown rice or quinoa

¼ cup sliced green olives

Directions:

1. Preheat oven to 400°.
2. Halve the peppers and remove the seeds, stem, and veins. Place them in a baking dish, cut sides up. Set aside.
3. In a large skillet over medium heat, brown the meat with the garlic, onion, and cumin.
4. Add the tomato sauce and continue to cook until the mixture is heated all the way through, about 3 minutes.
5. Remove the meat mixture from heat. Stir in the rice or quinoa and sliced olives.
6. Scoop equal amounts of the meat-and-rice mixture into each pepper half.
7. Bake until the peppers are soft, approximately 25 minutes.

Recipe tip:

Your holiday guests will love these! If you want, top them with your favorite cheese.

CRANBERRY SWEET POTATO BREAD

Serves 8

Ingredients:

¼ cup water

2 tablespoons ground flaxseed

1 medium sweet potato, diced

1 cup whole-grain or gluten-free flour

1 cup cornmeal

¼ cup raw sugar or stevia

4 teaspoons baking powder

1 teaspoon sea salt

1 cup rice, almond, or coconut milk

¼ cup olive oil

¼ cup maple syrup or agave syrup

½ cup dried cranberries

Directions:

1. Preheat oven to 425° and coat an 8 x 8-inch baking dish with nonstick cooking spray.
2. Bring the ¼ cup water to a boil in a small saucepan. Add the ground flaxseed and simmer until thickened, about 2 minutes. Set aside.
3. Place a steamer basket into a pan with water and bring to a boil. Add sweet potato. Steam until tender, approximately 15 minutes. Then remove sweet potato from pan.
4. Mash the sweet potato and set aside.
5. In a medium bowl, whisk together the flour, cornmeal, sugar or stevia, baking powder, and sea salt until fully mixed.
6. In a separate bowl, mix the wet ingredients: milk, olive oil, and maple or agave syrup. Add the ground flaxseed mixture from step 2.

7. Fold the wet ingredients into the dry ingredients, and then gently fold in the mashed sweet potato and dried cranberries to create the batter.

8. Pour the batter into the prepared baking pan and bake for 20 to 25 minutes, or until a toothpick inserted in the center comes out clean.

9. Let cool for 10 minutes.

Recipe tip:

Try using raisins instead of dried cranberries. This is sure to be another one of your holiday guests' favorites!

STUFF ME FULL TURKEY
Serves 12

Ingredients:

1 turkey, 10–15 pounds

4 sprigs rosemary

10 apples, cored and sliced in half

½ cup canola or sunflower oil

½ cup balsamic vinegar

1 tablespoon sea salt

1 tablespoon cinnamon

Directions:

1. To thaw a frozen turkey, place it in the refrigerator. (It takes about one day for every 4 to 5 pounds; a 15-pound bird needs 3 days.) Another method is to thaw the bird in a cold-water bath, changing the water every half hour. (This requires 30 minutes per pound—7½ hours for a 15-pound bird.)

2. When the turkey is fully thawed, preheat oven to 325°.

3. Remove the packet of giblets and the neck from the turkey's cavities.

4. Rinse the bird well (inside and outside) and pat dry with paper towels.

5. Place the turkey in a roasting pan, breast side up. Put rosemary in the large cavity of the bird, along with 2 apple halves.

6. Truss (tie legs together with string), then drizzle the bird with oil and balsamic vinegar, and sprinkle with salt and cinnamon.

7. Wedge remainder of apples around roasting pan to prop up the turkey evenly.

8. Place roasting pan in oven on lowest rack.

9. Roast 15 minutes per pound (a 15-pound turkey requires 3 hours and 45 minutes).

10. Check turkey with an instant-read thermometer to make sure it is fully cooked (the temperature should be 180° when inserted in the thickest part of the leg). Once the turkey is done, remove turkey from the oven and let it cool for 30 minutes before carving.

Recipe tip:

Substitute oranges for apples.

VEGGIE PIE

Serves 4 (in individual custard dishes)

Ingredients for pie filling:

1 large sweet potato, peeled and chopped into ½-inch pieces

1 large carrot, peeled and chopped

1 stalk celery, chopped

1 medium onion, chopped

⅓ cup fresh or frozen corn

1 large shiitake mushroom, chopped

¾ cup chopped broccoli florets

½ zucchini, chopped

⅓ cup fresh or frozen peas

4–6 garlic cloves, chopped fine

1 tablespoon whole-grain or gluten-free flour

2 cups vegetable broth or water

1 bay leaf

1 teaspoon fresh or dried oregano, or to taste

1 to 2 teaspoons sea salt

⅛ teaspoon black pepper, or to taste

1 pinch red pepper flakes

Directions for pie filling:

1. Sauté sweet potato, carrot, celery, onion, corn, mushroom, broccoli, zucchini, peas, and garlic in a skillet until tender crisp.
2. Whisk flour into broth or water and add to pot.
3. Add bay leaf, oregano, salt, black pepper, and red pepper flakes. Heat, stirring occasionally, until sauce is thickened and bubbling.
4. Remove from heat, discard the bay leaf, and divide the mixture among four custard dishes.

Ingredients for the top crust:

1½ cups whole-grain or gluten-free flour

¼ cup + 2 tablespoons butter

1 egg white

½ teaspoon salt

3 tablespoons canola or sunflower oil

3 tablespoons olive oil

1½ tablespoons apple cider vinegar

2½ tablespoons cold water

Directions for top crust:

1. Preheat oven to 350°.
2. In a large bowl, stir together flour, butter, egg white, and salt.
3. Add oils, apple cider vinegar, and water. Mix with a fork or your hands, forming the dough into a ball. If dough seems too dry, you can add a little more water.
4. Place the dough ball on a clean surface, dusted with flour. With a rolling pin, roll the dough into a ¼-inch thick sheet. Cut out circles slightly larger than the baking dishes.
5. Using a spatula, transfer your dough circles onto the top of your filled serving dishes. Gently press the dough with your finger all around the edge of each dish to seal the crust.
6. Brush the tops of the crust with a thin coat of olive oil, and bake for 15 to 25 minutes, until the crust is slightly cracked and a light golden brown color.
7. Let veggie pies cool for a few minutes and enjoy!

Recipe tip:

Try adding chicken or turkey for a more traditional potpie recipe.

PUMPKIN, SPICE, AND EVERYTHING NICE COOKIES

Makes about a dozen cookies

Ingredients:

8 ounces organic mashed pumpkin (canned or fresh)

1 small ripe banana, chopped

1½ teaspoons pumpkin pie spice

3 tablespoons agave syrup or honey

1 tablespoon raw sugar or stevia

¼ teaspoon sea salt, finely ground

2 cups organic raw whole rolled oats

3 tablespoons ground flaxseed

Directions:

1. Preheat the oven to 350°.
2. Coat a baking sheet with olive oil or canola oil cooking spray.
3. Combine pumpkin, banana, pumpkin pie spice, sweeteners, and sea salt in a large mixing bowl. Mix on high with a hand mixer until mostly smooth, about 2 minutes.
4. Using a large wooden spoon, fold in the oats and flaxseed until mixed well.
5. Form cookies using a tablespoon and bake for 12 to 16 minutes or until set.
6. Let cool 10 minutes before eating.

Recipe tip:

If you love chocolate, this recipe is also great with semisweet chocolate chips.

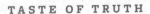

TASTE OF TRUTH

The best is yet to come—and when it does, our happiness will be everlasting.

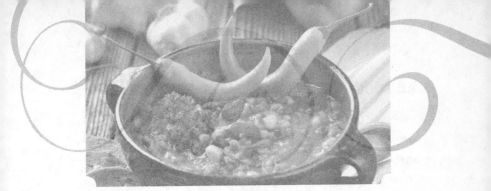

--| CHAPTER 7 |--

Craving God's Best for You

Spicy Food Recipes and Spicing Up Your Faith

I ONCE READ THAT cayenne pepper was good for weight loss. I'm one of those excessively compulsive people who believe that if a little is good, a lot must be better, so I decided to take half a bottle of cayenne pepper spicy seasoning and pour it into some tomato juice. Then I chugged it, hoping to be thin by the next morning.

Within twenty minutes of my spicy culinary experiment, I was rushed to an emergency room because my face had become so flushed and my blood pressure had gone through the roof. The medical staff had to give me a tranquilizer to calm me down and Benadryl for the allergic reaction.

You may be laughing right now, wondering what kind of woman I am to do something wacky like that. However, when we are craving spice in our lives, we can do some crazy things. Sadly, some of those things may even harm us and others.

Soul Food

. . . .

"Praise the LORD your God, who delights in you and has placed you on the throne as king to rule for him. Because God loves Israel and desires this kingdom to last forever, he has made you king over them so you can rule with justice and righteousness."

Then she gave the king a gift of 9,000 pounds of gold, great quantities of spices, and precious jewels. Never before had there been spices as fine as those the queen of Sheba gave to King Solomon.

2 CHRONICLES 9:8-9

Many times when you and I crave spice in our lives, we try to season ourselves with riches, when the Creator of the universe is just waiting for us to invite Him to pour His presence, peace, and power into our lives!

The Lord is waiting to season your life with lots of flavor and His favor. Consider the three ideas in the following New Life Recipes so that you may taste and see that your Lord can satisfy your craving like nothing else.

New Life Recipes

. . . .

1. GIVE IN

I will give you a new heart, and I will put a new spirit in you. I will take out your stony, stubborn heart and give you a tender, responsive heart.

EZEKIEL 36:26

Many times we are so set in our ways that we cannot see God's ways. He created us to crave spice in our lives, and He wants to take our hardened hearts and help us become who we crave to be. Take an honest inventory of your deepest desires. If you discover you want anything more than you want His will for your life, try a new spice I call "Giving In to Him." Then you will taste and see that the Lord is good.

2. GIVE IT AWAY

Jesus took the five loaves and two fish, looked up toward heaven, and blessed them. . . . They all ate as much as they wanted, and afterward, the disciples picked up twelve baskets of leftovers!

LUKE 9:16-17

A young boy came to eat lunch and listen to Jesus. Then he got so much more when he decided to give up all he had. Jesus took what the boy willingly gave away and fed the entire crowd—about five thousand men, not to mention the many women and children! Just think about the miracle that boy could have missed being a part of if he had kept his lunch for himself out of fear he would not have enough to eat. Nothing will do more to spice up your faith than to see God multiply what you're willing to give away.

3. GIVE IT UP

No one can take my life from me. I sacrifice it voluntarily. For I have the authority to lay it down when I want to and also to take it up again. For this is what my Father has commanded.

JOHN 10:18

When you think about Jesus giving up His life for us, it really puts all the things we think we can't give up in perspective, doesn't it?

If you want to add spice to your life, ask the Lord what He wants you to give up for your good and His glory.

POWER UP WITH PRAYER

Create in me a clean heart, O God.
Renew a loyal spirit within me.
Do not banish me from your presence,
and don't take your Holy Spirit from me.
PSALM 51:10-11

Dear God,
From this day forward I choose to give in to Your will and
to give away whatever You ask me to, as well as whatever is
getting in the way of my walk with You. I invite You now to
search my heart, so that through the power of the Holy Spirit,
I will see what I need to do to taste and see Your goodness
again. Amen.

FOOD TRUTH

No food . . . is more flavorful than life in Christ.

Spicy Food Recipes

Who says healthy food needs to taste boring and bland? Add a little zip to your next meal with one of the following recipes.

FANTASTIC FIERY CHICKEN
Serves 4–6

Ingredients:

2 tablespoons tomato paste

1½ teaspoons water

½ teaspoon olive oil

½ teaspoon minced garlic

½ teaspoon chipotle chili powder

½ teaspoon fresh oregano, chopped

4 boneless chicken breasts

Directions for marinade:

1. Blend together the tomato paste, water, and oil in a small bowl.
2. Add garlic, chili powder, and oregano. Mix well.
3. Using a brush, spread the marinade on both sides of the chicken breasts and refrigerate overnight.

Directions for cooking chicken:

1. Prepare a charcoal or gas grill and lightly coat the grill's cooking rack or grid with nonstick cooking spray. Position it 4 to 6 inches from the heat source.
2. Place chicken on grill and cook thoroughly, about 15 to 20 minutes.

Recipe tip:

If you really love hot spice, take some jalapeños and squeeze the juice on the chicken while it's cooking!

HOT CABBAGE

Serves 2–4

Ingredients:

1½ pounds red cabbage, cored, quartered, and shredded

1 medium onion, chopped

1 tart apple, cored and chopped

1 garlic clove, crushed

1 teaspoon ground cinnamon

¼ teaspoon ground cloves

1 teaspoon cumin seed

1 tablespoon cayenne pepper

2 tablespoons red wine vinegar

2 teaspoons red pepper flakes

½ teaspoon ground nutmeg, or to taste

1 tablespoon jalapeño juice, optional

½ cup water

Directions:

1. In a large pot, stir all the ingredients together, mixing thoroughly.
2. Cover and cook over medium heat, stirring frequently until the vegetables are tender, about 1 hour.
3. Add more water as needed during the cooking process to prevent the mixture from going dry or burning.
4. Transfer to a serving bowl and serve either warm or cold.

Recipe tip:

Serve as a side dish or add meat for a heartier entrée. This is also a great side dish to a soup!

SPICY SQUASH

Serves 2–4

Ingredients:

1 spaghetti squash, cut in half and seeds scraped out

4 tablespoons olive oil, divided

Salt and pepper

4 cloves garlic, minced

1 zucchini, halved and sliced

1 teaspoon red pepper flakes

Fresh chopped herbs, to taste

Directions:

1. Preheat oven to 400°.
2. Rub about 1 tablespoon of olive oil inside each squash half, and season to taste with salt and pepper.
3. Place each piece of squash, skin side up, on a baking tray.
4. Bake for 45 minutes.
5. Remove the squash from the oven and allow it to cool slightly. Be careful, as the skin will be very hot.
6. Using a fork, pull the spaghetti-like strands of squash pulp from the skin into a mixing bowl.
7. Place 2 tablespoons of olive oil in a skillet and add the garlic, zucchini, and red pepper flakes. Heat together on medium-high heat for about 1 minute.
8. Pour the zucchini mixture over the squash and stir it in. Then add chopped fresh herbs and mix again.

Recipe tip:

Treat this like spaghetti. Add a zesty red sauce or Parmesan to make it extra delicious.

AREN'T WE TENDER, PORK TENDERLOIN

Serves 4

Ingredients:

½ teaspoon freshly grated or ground ginger

½ teaspoon garlic powder

½ teaspoon onion powder

½ teaspoon cayenne pepper

1 teaspoon ground cinnamon

½ teaspoon ground cloves

2 teaspoons firmly packed brown sugar

¾ teaspoon sea salt, divided

½ teaspoon freshly ground black pepper

1 pork tenderloin, about 1 pound, trimmed of fat

1½ cups raw honey

1 teaspoon tomato paste

2 teaspoons white vinegar

1 tablespoon red pepper flakes

Directions:

1. Prepare a hot fire in a charcoal grill or heat a gas grill or oven broiler to medium-high temperature, about 400°.
2. In a small bowl, combine the ginger, garlic powder, onion powder, cayenne pepper, cinnamon, cloves, brown sugar, ½ teaspoon of the sea salt, and the black pepper to make a rub.
3. Place the meat in the bowl and rub the spice mixture over the pork. Let stand for 15 minutes.
4. In another small bowl, combine the honey, tomato paste, vinegar, red pepper flakes, and the remaining ¼ teaspoon of sea salt. Stir to blend. Set aside.

5. Place the pork on the grill rack or broiler pan. Grill or broil, turning several times, until browned, about 3 minutes on each side.

6. Move to a cooler part of the grill or reduce the heat. Continue cooking for about 14 to 16 minutes. Baste with the honey-vinegar glaze and continue cooking until the pork is slightly pink inside and an instant-read thermometer inserted into the thickest part reads 160°.

7. Move pork to a cutting board. Let stand for 5 minutes before slicing.

Recipe tip:
This is a great recipe to make when guests come for the holidays!

FIRE CHILI

Serves 8

Ingredients:

1½ cups coarsely chopped
    onion

1 cup chopped red bell
    pepper

1 cup chopped green bell
    pepper

3 cloves garlic, minced

¾ cup chopped celery

¾ cup chopped carrot

3 jalapeños, sliced

1 tablespoon chili powder

1½ cups quartered fresh
    mushrooms

1 cup cubed zucchini

1 can (11 ounces) whole kernel
    corn, undrained

1 tablespoon ground cumin

1 can (15 ounces) chickpeas,
    drained and rinsed

1 can (15 ounces) black beans,
    drained and rinsed

1 can (15 ounces) diced
    or whole tomatoes,
    undrained, or 1 cup fresh
    diced tomatoes

1½ teaspoons dried oregano

1½ teaspoons dried basil

½ teaspoon cayenne pepper

Directions:

1. Coat a large saucepan with nonstick cooking spray. Add onion, red bell pepper, green bell pepper, garlic, celery, carrot, jalapeños, and chili powder. Cook over medium heat until vegetables are soft.
2. Add mushrooms and zucchini. Cook for 4 minutes.
3. Add corn, ground cumin, chickpeas, black beans, tomatoes with juice, oregano, basil, and cayenne pepper. Bring to a boil, then reduce heat to medium-low. Cover and simmer for 20 minutes, stirring occasionally.

Recipe tip:

If this still isn't spicy enough for you, add some red pepper flakes.

GARLIC SPICED CHICKEN
Serves 4–6

Ingredients:

3 cloves garlic, crushed

1 teaspoon fresh grated ginger

½ teaspoon cayenne pepper

⅓ cup hoisin sauce

3 tablespoons low-sodium soy sauce or Bragg Liquid Aminos

¼ cup red wine vinegar

1 teaspoon sesame oil

12 chicken drumsticks

2 teaspoons brown sugar

½ teaspoon whole-grain or gluten-free flour

½ teaspoon water

Directions:

1. Combine garlic, ginger, cayenne pepper, hoisin sauce, soy sauce or Bragg Liquid Aminos, red wine vinegar, and sesame oil in a large bowl. Mix well to make a marinade.
2. Add chicken to marinade and turn to coat all sides. Cover and refrigerate for 3 hours or overnight.
3. Drain chicken, reserving marinade.
4. Heat a grill or broiler pan to medium heat, about 350°. Grill chicken until fully cooked and browned to your liking.
5. Blend brown sugar, flour, and water in a pan over medium-high heat. Stir in reserved marinade, and continue stirring until mixture boils and thickens. Serve sauce with chicken.

Recipe tip:

This chicken dish is delicious served over brown rice.

HOMEMADE BARBECUE SAUCE

Makes a small bowl of sauce

Ingredients:

½ cup water

1½ cups tomato sauce

½ cup red wine vinegar

1 tablespoon low-sodium soy sauce or Bragg Liquid Aminos

½ teaspoon hot sauce

1 cup agave syrup or honey

2½ tablespoons dry mustard

2 teaspoons paprika

2 teaspoons salt

1½ teaspoons black pepper

Directions:

1. Combine water, tomato sauce, vinegar, soy sauce or Bragg Liquid Aminos, and hot sauce in a blender.
2. Season mixture with remaining ingredients; blend until smooth.

TASTE OF TRUTH

His power displayed through you will spice up everyone else's faith.

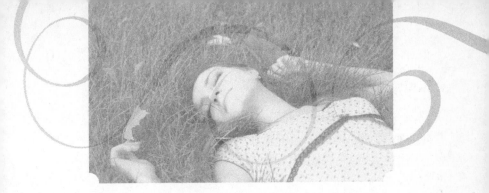

CHAPTER 8

Craving Real Refreshment

Delicious Drinks and Hydration for Your Soul

I WASN'T RAISED a Christian, and I did not give my life to the Lord until I was twenty-four. I had much time to live in the world and act like the world. During my early years, everyone I knew seemed to be driven by a desire for pleasure.

After I became a Christian, I watched most believers try to walk out their faith according to other people's expectations—almost as if they were Christian clones. Neither approach—living for pleasure as a nonbeliever or without a unique purpose as a believer—seemed to offer refreshment to me or anybody else. I assumed everyone's soul was as severely dehydrated as mine.

Today I know the Lord and understand that He created me with a distinct purpose in mind, but I still sometimes find myself seeking refreshment from things, people, or pleasure. It's not that we cannot find temporary refreshment from those three things, but they will not quench our thirst or cure the craving of our hearts and souls.

Soul Food

. . . .

Then times of refreshment will come from the presence of the Lord, and he will again send you Jesus, your appointed Messiah.

ACTS 3:20

Have you ever jumped into a lukewarm pool on a hot summer day? When you're overly warm, it's pretty disappointing to land in what feels like bathwater. No matter how many times you jump in or how long you stay in, you won't be cooled and refreshed.

Sometimes we crave refreshment because our faith feels lukewarm. We don't feel cold, and we don't feel hot. We're just going through the motions. Jesus said He came to give us life and all it has to offer. So how can we truly live the abundant life He gave His own life for? We need the real deal, and that is not easily found when we have settled for an artificial connection with God and one another.

For example, we crave refreshment in our relationships, yet texting and e-mail have become the new ways to connect. Don't get me wrong: it's not that I don't love text messaging my friends and family, but I know nothing replaces the heart-to-heart connection that comes when you spend quality time sharing your heart and looking into a friend's or family member's eyes.

We crave a breath of fresh air, but we don't allow ourselves to stop for a moment and breathe in the blessings that surround us. We crave peace for our minds, but we won't turn off the TV long enough to clear our minds of the junk we watch and simply be still before the Lord.

Refreshment is found in the simple things: a walk in a park or by a river, a good talk with a friend, a quiet afternoon, a Sunday nap in the chaise lounge or hammock in the yard. . . . Take a moment and think about the things that refresh you. Then read the three New Life Recipes that follow to help you find the refreshment you are craving.

New Life Recipes
· ·

1. REFRESH OTHERS

The generous will prosper; those who refresh others will themselves
be refreshed.

PROVERBS 11:25

When we're worn out and weary, how many times do we look to our
loved ones to refresh us? Then, when they don't give us the refreshment
we crave, we are disappointed in them.

All along God is saying, "Come to Me to get refreshment. Then go
out and be My representative and refresh others." The Lord promises us
in Proverbs that if we refresh others, we ourselves will be refreshed by
Him. Let's refresh those we love today!

2. LIE DOWN

He lets me rest in green meadows;
*   he leads me beside peaceful streams.*

PSALM 23:2

When you feel like your soul is dying of thirst and you have nothing
left to give, stop everything and be still. What you're craving is to be
filled up by the Holy Spirit. It's only when you sit at His feet—turning
off your phone and computer, putting down your to-do list—and allow
Him to pour His loving and living water over you that you will find the
refreshment you crave.

Don't underestimate the power of being still in His presence.

3. LIVE THIS DAY

This is the day the LORD has made.
*   We will rejoice and be glad in it.*

PSALM 118:24

97

We deprive ourselves of much-needed refreshment and burn out when we don't live for today. Too often our minds are in the next place we need to be or on the next thing we need to do. As a result, we don't feel satisfied; we feel frustrated. If we are not careful, we will miss those treasured moments that could refresh us.

If you're craving a breath of life, try to breathe in the moment. That means taking time to check in with whoever is standing in front of you today. As you do, you will find new refreshment.

POWER UP WITH PRAYER

> *He satisfies the thirsty*
> *and fills the hungry with good things.*
> PSALM 107:9

Dear God,
Your Word says that You satisfy the thirsty and fill the hungry
with good things. I am thirsty for Your presence in my life,
and I ask You to fill me up once again so I can fill others
up. Help me be still long enough to drink in Your goodness.
Amen.

FOOD TRUTH

**No food . . . refreshes
like God's Word.**

Refreshing Drink Recipes

For real refreshment on a hot summer day or after a hard workout, try whipping up one of the following cool drinks.

WATERMELON LEMONADE
Serves 8

Ingredients:

10 to 12 pounds seedless watermelon, cut up

4 tablespoons freshly squeezed lemon juice

2 tablespoons raw sugar or stevia

Directions:

1. Puree watermelon in batches in a blender. Transfer to large pitcher.
2. Mix in remaining ingredients.
3. Chill and serve for a deliciously refreshing drink!

Recipe tip:

Great for kids or yourself on a hot summer day. You can also create healthy frozen ice pops with this recipe.

STRAWBERRY LEMONADE

Serves 2–4

Ingredients:

2 cups frozen strawberries

2 cups peeled, seeded lemon, cut up

1 peeled, seeded orange, cut up

1 or 2 packets of stevia

2 cups crushed ice

1 to 2 cups water

1 lemon, peeled, seeded, and cut into 4 slices for garnish

Directions:

1. Place all ingredients in blender and mix for 1 to 2 minutes, until smooth.
2. Garnish each glass with a lemon slice for extra tang.

Recipe tip:

Replace the strawberries with raspberries to make raspberry lemonade. You can also freeze the liquid and make ice pops.

POMEGRANATE PUNCH

Serves 2–4

Ingredients:

8 pomegranate tea bags

2 cups hot water

3 cups pomegranate juice

1 tablespoon raw sugar or stevia

Directions:

1. Brew pomegranate tea in hot water, according to the package directions, then let the tea cool for 15 minutes.
2. Mix pomegranate juice and sugar or stevia in pitcher.
3. Add cooled tea. Pour into glasses with ice and serve.

Recipe tip:

You can also blend this with ice to make a smoothie, or freeze to make ice pops.

THAT'S THE RASPBERRIES SMOOTHIE

Serves 2–3

Ingredients:

1 cup plain nonfat yogurt

1½ cups frozen raspberries

1 teaspoon vanilla extract

½ cup vanilla coconut milk

½ cup honey

1½ cups ice (more if needed)

Directions:

Blend all ingredients together to desired consistency. Pour into glasses and enjoy!

Recipe tip:

You can also freeze this into ice pops for a healthy, refreshing snack.

FRUIT SPRITZER
Serves 1–2

Ingredients:

½ cup naturally sweetened raspberry or cranberry juice, chilled

1 cup sparkling mineral water, chilled

1 lime, cut into 4 wedges

Directions:

1. Stir the raspberry or cranberry juice and mineral water together.
2. Pour into ice-filled glasses. Before serving, add lime wedges.

Recipe tip:

You can add any flavor packet of Emergen-C for some added vitamin C and antioxidants.

GINGERLY PEACHY KEEN SMOOTHIE

Serves 2–4

Ingredients:

1 cup plain low-fat yogurt

1 tablespoon fresh grated ginger

1 teaspoon vanilla extract

½ cup fat-free cottage cheese

⅓ cup honey

4 large peaches, sliced

Directions:

1. Combine ingredients in blender and mix until smooth. Pour into glasses and serve.

Recipe tip:

Try this with mangoes for another delicious smoothie.

FROZEN HONEY COLADA SMOOTHIE

Serves 4

Ingredients:

4 teaspoons honey

1 cup pineapple

2 cups coconut milk

4 cups ice cubes

Directions:

Combine all ingredients in blender, and mix for 30 seconds.

Recipe tip:

If you love coconut, top off your drink with shredded coconut for some extra taste.

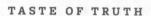

TASTE OF TRUTH

Life is not measured by the number of breaths we take but by the moments that take our breath away! (Author unknown)

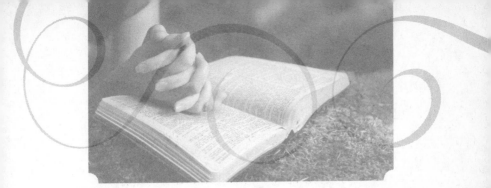

---| CHAPTER 9 |---

Craving Fortifying Faith

Raw Food Recipes and Getting Real with God

ONCE AS I WAS being interviewed live on a Christian television program, I noticed a large, very loud fly buzzing around the set of the studio. It kept landing on the bald head of the show's host, who was sitting across from me.

I did everything I could to pretend I did not see that fly—until it flew into the host's mouth. Though he continued to ignore what was real—the bug he was choking on—and went on interviewing me, I was not as good an actress as he was an actor. I finally broke out in laughter; needless to say, the show got very real at that moment.

I think sometimes we are so afraid to talk about what's really going on that we forget how freeing it is for everyone around us when we get real with one another. Of course, it's even more important that we get real with God.

Soul Food

. . . .

> *O Lord, how long will you forget me?*
> > *Forever?*
> *How long will you look the other way? . . .*
> > *Turn and answer me, O Lord my God!*
> *Restore the sparkle to my eyes, or*
> > *I will die.*

PSALM 13:1, 3

There was nothing artificial about King David's relationship with the Lord. If you read the book of Psalms, you will see that David had a very real and authentic relationship with God. David was not perfect, but he was desperate for God and not afraid to admit it! His desperation led God to give David a very distinct description: "a man after my own heart" (Acts 13:22).

In the deepest part of every man and woman is a craving for real faith. Today, due to so many false teachings and fallen leaders, many people's faith has been fractured. But that doesn't stop our craving to find the true and living God.

Remember that man is *not* God, so if a *man* or *woman* (your pastor, father, mother, boss, or friend) has sinned against God or you, please be careful not to lose your faith because of that person's actions.

That means, first of all, that we have to get real and recognize that we live in a fallen world with imperfect people. If we are ever going to find real faith, it won't be in a man—it will be in the true and living God who designed us to have a real relationship with Him.

If you're craving closeness with your heavenly Father, then I invite you to join me in finding real faith cures to connect your heart in a very real way to the one true and very real God!

New Life Recipes

1. DON'T LOOK TO OTHERS

Dear friends, do not believe everyone who claims to speak by the Spirit. You must test them to see if the spirit they have comes from God. For there are many false prophets in the world.

    1 JOHN 4:1

God warns us not to believe everything we see or hear from people. He tells us that not everyone who says he or she is a Christian represents God.

If you're craving a real faith relationship with the Lord, it won't be found by looking to others; it will be found by looking to God. He promises that if you seek Him with all your heart, you will find Him. If you're really craving more of God, commit yourself to praying and seeking a real relationship with Him. Then you will find the real faith your heart longs for.

2. DON'T PLAY FAITH GAMES

But I fear that somehow your pure and undivided devotion to Christ will be corrupted, just as Eve was deceived by the cunning ways of the serpent.

    2 CORINTHIANS 11:3

God loved Eve and gave her the opportunity to be blessed in every way. However, she caved in to her curiosity, hoping it would satisfy her heart's desire to know the truth. In that moment of deception, she played a game in her own mind and allowed the enemy to convince her that God didn't really mean what He said. By acting on that craving, she sinned. Adam soon followed, and their actions were the cause of death for every one of us.

Don't make Adam and Eve's mistake. If you want a real relationship with God, you must crave obeying Him more than anything else. God is who He says He is, and He will do what He says He will do. Let's get real with Him and get our hearts right so we can receive His blessing.

3. DON'T LIVE BY SIGHT

For we live by believing and not by seeing.

2 CORINTHIANS 5:7

Prior to finding Christ in my midtwenties, I saw a lot of horrible things, which made it difficult for me to live by faith and not by sight. I craved real peace and a real relationship with God, yet somehow I could not understand why bad things happen to good people and why unjust things happen in the world that God created.

Today I understand that faith is all about living by what I know to be true in the Word, not by what I see around me. I now understand that I cannot control others' actions, but I can control my reactions to the world around me by the power of God.

Be real with God. Let Him know your fears and your frustrations. Tell Him when you cannot find Him, and ask Him to make Himself real to you. Then you will begin to see the invisible God become visible to you and through you.

POWER UP WITH PRAYER

[Jesus said,] "The time is coming—indeed it's here now—when you will be scattered, each one going his own way, leaving me alone. Yet I am not alone because the Father is with me. I have told you all this so that you may have peace in me. Here on earth you will have many trials and sorrows. But take heart, because I have overcome the world."

JOHN 16:32-33

Dear God,
It is hard to find You in a world that is filled with pain,
problems, and persecution. I am getting real with You and
letting You know that I need You to reveal Yourself to me in
a personal way today. I love You, and I want and crave more
of You. Amen.

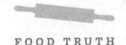

FOOD TRUTH

No food . . . can control you
without your permission.

Raw Food Recipes

The benefits of going raw are extensive, particularly since so many of our foods are pumped with preservatives and additives. Going raw eliminates the need to wonder and worry about what you are really eating. Raw food is delicious, and eating it will make you feel amazing.

RAW FOOD RANCH DRESSING
Serves 2–4

Ingredients:

¼–½ cup almonds, soaked in water overnight

2 cloves garlic, minced

Juice of 1 lemon

¾ cup canola or sunflower oil

¼ teaspoon kelp granules or sea salt

A touch of honey

Directions:

1. Drain and rinse the almonds.
2. In blender, add almonds to all other ingredients and mix thoroughly. The dressing should be nice and thick.

Recipe tip:

Almond skins will turn the dressing brown. If you want the dressing to be white, you can blanch the almonds by putting them in boiling water for 30 seconds. After 30 seconds, slowly add cool water until the water is warm. Peel off the almond skins with your fingers. This is a great dip for any fresh veggies.

MUSHROOM SOUP
Serves 4–6

Ingredients:

2 tablespoons olive oil

1½ cups sliced fresh mushrooms

1 red onion, diced

2 carrots, grated

1 tablespoon minced garlic

8 cups vegetable broth

3 cups cooked pearl barley

1 teaspoon sea salt

Directions:

1. Heat olive oil in a large soup pot and add mushrooms, onion, carrots, and garlic. Cook for 5 minutes.
2. Add vegetable broth, barley, and sea salt. Simmer for about 40 minutes over low heat.
3. Serve in bowls and enjoy.

Recipe tip:

Feel free to add any other vegetables that you love to this recipe—celery leaves or kale would be fantastic!

TASTY RAW FOOD TACOS

Serves 4–6

Ingredients:

8 ounces salsa

1 cup cashews

1 cup sunflower seeds

8–12 corn or gluten-free tortillas

1½ cups diced cooked chicken

½ red onion, diced

1 cup cooked black beans

2 ripe tomatoes, diced

1 avocado, diced

1 mango, diced

Directions:

1. Blend together salsa, cashews, and sunflower seeds to a pastelike consistency.
2. Lay tortillas flat and spread with the salsa/cashew/sunflower seed mixture. Top with the chicken, onion, black beans, tomatoes, avocado, and mango. Fold over like a taco, and enjoy!

Recipe tip:

Dress up your tacos with organic lettuce, or if you're feeling really brave, substitute cabbage leaves for the corn tortillas for an all-raw meal!

GOOD-FOR-YOU GREENS SOUP

Serves 2–4

Ingredients:

1 cup fresh diced tomato

½ cup water

2 cups spinach

½ avocado

½ cup chopped broccoli

1 teaspoon fresh minced garlic or garlic powder

2 tablespoons freshly squeezed or bottled lemon juice

1 tablespoon olive oil

Directions:

1. Place all the ingredients in a blender, and mix until smooth.
2. Pour mixture into a saucepan, and heat 5 to 10 minutes, stirring as needed. Taste to make sure it has the flavor you want. You can add water if soup is too thick.

Recipe tip:

A great side dish to this soup would be sweet potato fries, made fresh in your oven!

RAW MANGO PUDDING

Serves 2–4

Ingredients:

4 cups frozen mango chunks

1 fresh peach or nectarine

1 ripe banana

2 dates

1 passion fruit

1 tablespoon raw sugar or stevia

4 strawberries

Directions:

1. Chop all of the fruit.
2. Mix chopped fruit in the blender until smooth. Add ice if pudding is too thin.

Recipe tip:

This is a great party recipe, and it's also great for kids. Take some to work in a Tupperware container for a fun snack. It will keep in the fridge for up to three days.

FRESH CORN SALAD
Serves 2–4

Ingredients for salad:

2 cups fresh corn, cut from the cob

½ red onion, diced

¾ cup diced red, orange, and/or yellow bell peppers

1 avocado, diced

1 tomato, diced

1 cup cooked black beans

½ cup diced mild green chilies

Ingredients for dressing:

Juice of 1 lemon (about ¼ cup)

Juice of 1 lime (about ¼ cup)

1–2 garlic cloves, minced

½ bunch cilantro, chopped fine

4 ounces salsa

Directions:

1. Mix all salad ingredients together.
2. Mix all dressing ingredients together.
3. Mix salad with dressing and serve.

Recipe tip:

Add raw honey or agave syrup to the dressing mix for a sweeter taste to this salad.

MINT PEAR SALAD

Serves 2–4

Ingredients for salad:

1 head romaine lettuce

1 avocado, diced

2 pears, diced

½ cup slivered almonds

½ cup dried cranberries

Ingredients for mint dressing:

1 small bunch fresh mint

1½ tablespoons honey

Juice of 1 lemon

¾ cup low-fat or Healthy Mayonnaise (see page 21)

Directions:

1. Mix salad ingredients in a large bowl.
2. Mix dressing ingredients.
3. Mix dressing with salad, serve, and enjoy!

Recipe tip:

This dressing can be stored in the fridge for up to three days. The mint dressing works on any of your favorite salads or as a dip for fresh fruit. If you don't want to eat this completely raw, add diced cooked chicken breast for protein.

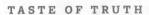

TASTE OF TRUTH

**Get real with God, and
He will become real to you.**

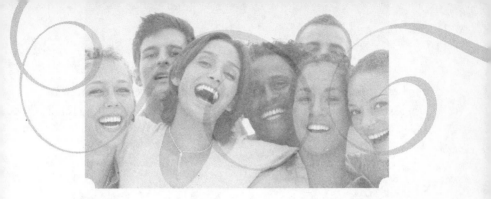

---| CHAPTER 10 |---

Craving Fun and Laughter

Fun Party Food and Fun Faith Ideas

WHEN I WAS IN HIGH SCHOOL, my friends referred to me as the life of the party—so much so that they told me they could not go through a weekend without me to entertain them.

Unfortunately for them, I was one of those teenagers who never cleaned her room—the only way my parents could motivate me to clean was to ground me until my room was tidy again. Many times I opted to stay home in my dirty room. Believe it or not, since I was their entertainment, my friends would often come to my home and clean my room for me so I could go out and have fun with them.

Looking back, that probably wasn't the best training for me as a young woman. Even today, though I love having a clean house, I would prefer to have someone else clean for me. My point is not about cleaning or getting others to do things for us; it is that while God does want us to have fun, He is a faithful Father who loves us so much that He wants our hearts to crave clean fun so we don't have to live with regrets. In other words, He wants us to recognize that a moment of pleasure is not worth a lifetime of pain.

Soul Food
· ·

Whether you eat or drink, or whatever you do, do it all for the glory of God.

I CORINTHIANS 10:31

All my life I have loved making people laugh. After I became a Christian, I didn't realize that God would use that gift to bring people closer to Him. Like many people, I had bought into the lie that to walk by faith means we cannot have fun and that craving fun is somehow a sin. Yet the Bible says that a merry heart makes the body healthy and that laughter can be medicine to our souls.

Fun can be a good thing when we crave it in a way that draws us closer to God and offers true joy to others. It's time for us to show the world that faith is a good thing that brings much peace, power, and pleasure into our lives.

If you're craving some fun, I invite you to try the following New Life Recipes, which I believe will bring some real joy back into your life.

New Life Recipes
· ·

1. WATCH CHRISTIAN OR CLEAN COMEDY

A cheerful heart is good medicine, but a broken spirit saps a person's strength.

PROVERBS 17:22

Laughter is a gift from God, and a cheerful heart is medicine to the soul. We don't have to watch inappropriate things to laugh; there are many amazing comedians who know how to help us laugh at life and ourselves without dishonoring God.

May I suggest a few sources of good, clean laughter: Anita Renfroe, Chonda Pierce, Brian Regan, Mark Lowry, and Bill Cosby.

For other ideas, use Google to search for "Christian comedians." Go on—allow yourself to laugh again.

2. READ A HUMOROUS CHRISTIAN BOOK OR BLOG

For the despondent, every day brings trouble; for the happy heart, life is a continual feast.

PROVERBS 15:15

Fun may be lacking in your life because of what you read. I invite you to look at the variety of amazing Christian books and blogs available that will bring you joy and laughter. They will also offer you some great life lessons that will draw you closer to God. Jonathan Acuff, Charlene Ann Baumbich, Jen Hatmaker, and Matt Mikalatos are just a few of the Christian authors who will keep you laughing.

I know that what we read truly impacts the way we think and feel, so treat yourself by reading and feeding your mind with the goodness of God found in His Word and through His people who write about the Good News.

3. HOST A "HIS PRINCESS" PARTY

You are royal priests, a holy nation, God's very own possession. As a result, you can show others the goodness of God, for he called you out of the darkness into his wonderful light.

I PETER 2:9

Consider hosting a princess party for grown-ups. Personalize the invitation with a Scripture about being a daughter of the King. Have the women dress in purple. Give each one of your guests a crown and a ribbon to wear across her body, perhaps a banner that says "daughter of the King." You can also have the women bring clothes they no longer wear and do a clothing exchange. Play upbeat Christian praise music and serve some of the great party food found in this chapter. It will be a great witness and a wonderful time!

POWER UP WITH PRAYER

You will show me the way of life,
*   granting me the joy of your presence*
and the pleasures of living with you forever.
PSALM 16:11

Dear God,
I am fighting to find joy in my life; I want my faith walk to
reflect Your glory and joy. Please help me to laugh again and
to embrace life in a whole new way! Show me a clean kind
of fun that brings honor to You and joy to others. I want a
merry heart that will become medicine to my soul. Amen.

FOOD TRUTH

No food . . . brings as much fun as glorifying God with your body.

Party Food Recipes

If you are planning to serve fun and festive finger foods and dips at your next get-together, try one or more of the following recipes.

ISLAND SNACK
Serves 2

Ingredients:

2 large ripe bananas

2 tablespoons natural cocoa powder

2 tablespoons shredded coconut

Directions:

Peel bananas and cut them in half, roll each half in cocoa powder, and sprinkle with shredded coconut.

Recipe tip:

What a great recipe for when you're having a party and want some fun finger foods! Cut the bananas into bite-size pieces before rolling them in cocoa powder and coconut. These will keep for one day in the fridge but are best the day they are made.

CREAMY FRUIT SALAD

Serves 1–2

Ingredients for salad:

Whatever fruits you choose

Directions for salad:

1. Wash or peel fruits and cut into bite-size pieces.
2. Mix fruits in large bowl.

Ingredients for cream:

1 can (13–16 ounces) unsweetened coconut milk

¼ cup agave syrup

½ teaspoon vanilla extract

Directions for cream:

1. In blender, mix ingredients until thick and smooth. If there is not enough cream for the amount of people you are serving, simply keep doubling the recipe until you have enough.
2. Drizzle cream on top of each salad portion and serve.

Recipe tip:

Try the cream in a fruit smoothie or as a dip with pretzels for a salty-sweet snack. This recipe will keep for two to three days in the fridge.

MUSHROOM DIP

Serves 4–6

Ingredients:

5 cups mushrooms

3 tablespoons butter

½ cup coconut milk

1 teaspoon onion powder

1 pinch sea salt

Directions:

1. Cook mushrooms and butter in skillet until tender.
2. In blender, mix all ingredients until thick and smooth.
3. Spoon into bowl and serve.

Recipe tip:

Great with pita chips, tortilla chips, or as a side dip for meats at any of your parties. Your guests will absolutely love this dip!

HUMMUS WITH ROASTED RED PEPPER AND TOMATO

Fills a medium-size bowl

Ingredients:

2 (15.5 ounces) cans low-sodium garbanzo beans or 2 cups almonds, soaked in water overnight

½ cup tahini

1 large garlic clove, minced

3 tablespoons freshly squeezed or bottled lemon juice

½ teaspoon sea salt

½ cup chopped red bell peppers

¼ cup chopped sun-dried tomatoes

Directions:

1. If using almonds, grind nuts using a blender or hand mixer. (It helps to chop the almonds first.) Set chopped almonds aside in bowl.
2. Add all other ingredients into the blender and mix until smooth. Add almonds or garbanzo beans. Add water if needed to get the consistency you desire.
3. Place in bowl and serve to guests.

Recipe tip:

Serve with whole-grain or gluten-free crackers or pita chips.

VEGETABLE SLAW
Serves 8

Ingredients:

¼ teaspoon sea salt

¼ teaspoon coarsely ground pepper

1 tablespoon prepared horseradish

2 teaspoons celery seed

½ cup low-fat or Healthy Mayonnaise (see page 21)

½ cup low-fat sour cream

1 cup diced celery

1 medium green onion, diced fine

1 small head green cabbage, shredded (about 2 cups)

1 small jicama, shredded

1 small head red cabbage, shredded

Cilantro, to taste

Directions:

1. Combine sea salt, pepper, horseradish, celery seed, mayonnaise, and sour cream in a small bowl.
2. Mix remaining ingredients in a large bowl, pour dressing over the vegetables, and toss gently to mix. Serve immediately.

Recipe tip:

This is such a delicious party salad and a great side dish for any meat. Consider using Vegenaise instead of mayonnaise if you want a slaw lower in fat.

ROLLOVER TURKEY

Serves approximately 12 to 15

Ingredients:

1 pound smoked turkey, sliced thick

1 tub soft cream cheese

1 jar pickle spears

Directions:

1. Take a turkey slice, spread cream cheese thinly on one side, place pickle spear on an edge of the turkey slice, and roll the turkey around the pickle.
2. Cut the turkey rolls in halves or thirds, and stick a toothpick through each piece to secure it.
3. Repeat with each turkey slice until you have enough.

Recipe tip:

Try using miso-flavored mayonnaise instead of cream cheese for some extra-flavorful rolls!

HONEY-BAKED ALMOND BRITTLE

Serves 4

Ingredients:

¼ cup honey

1 cup almonds

Dash sea salt

Directions:

1. Preheat oven to 350°.
2. Heat honey in microwave for 30 seconds.
3. In a bowl, pour honey over the almonds and mix evenly so every almond is coated.
4. Coat cookie sheet with nonstick spray, spread almonds on cookie sheet, and sprinkle with sea salt.
5. Bake at 350° for 15 minutes. Let cool, and enjoy!

Recipe tip:

This is a great topping for chocolate or vanilla ice cream. Your guests will love this unique brittle!

TASTE OF TRUTH

Fun happens when our faith becomes bigger than our fears and frustration.

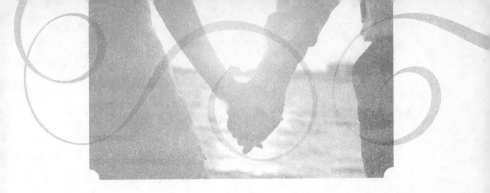

CHAPTER 11

Craving Romance and Unconditional Love

Romantic Recipes for Two and Marinating Your Marriage

I LOVE CHICK FLICKS. I love the romance and the heart connection seen on the big screen between a man and a woman. Too many times we are told that a Christian marriage does not need romance, and we are made to feel guilty for craving it. However, never before has an upcoming generation so needed to see love expressed romantically between a husband and wife.

Our heavenly Father understands a woman's desire to feel loved and romanced by her man. He also knows the passion that burns inside a man for a woman. After all, He created that kind of love!

Soul Food

. . . .

> *You are beautiful, my darling,*
> *beautiful beyond words.*
> *Your eyes are like doves*
> *behind your veil.*
> *Your hair falls in waves. . . .*
> *Your lips are like scarlet ribbon;*
> *your mouth is inviting.*
> *Your cheeks are like rosy pomegranates*
> *behind your veil.*
> SONG OF SONGS 4:1, 3

The passage above is just one small section from the Song of Songs, which records an extremely expressive and romantic conversation between a man and a woman who are married. And yes, it is recorded in the bestselling book of all time . . . the Bible.

I am convinced after reading the Song of Songs that romantic expressions of love between a man and woman do not simply hold them together. Just as important, they speak to a world that is watching how we love one another. Nothing brings more glory to God than when a husband and a wife love each other in the way God intended. If you're ready to marinate your marriage with mutual devotion, join me as I offer a few suggestions in the following New Life Recipes.

New Life Recipes

. . . .

1. FLIRT WITH YOUR HUSBAND

> *You are so handsome, my love,*
> *pleasing beyond words!*
> *The soft grass is our bed;*

fragrant cedar branches are the beams of our house,
and pleasant smelling firs are the rafters.
SONG OF SONGS 1:16-17

Okay, I know it may sound crazy to suggest that you flirt with your husband. But you probably flirted with him to get his attention, so why did you ever stop? Flirting with each other will stimulate your love and attraction. And it will keep you thinking about each other when someone else tries to flirt with either one of you.

Write little love notes, talk about fun things you can do together, and laugh at your husband's jokes (even if you don't think they're funny). Humor is a great way to flirt with one another, and it will bring joy and laughter to your relationship.

2. RELAX WITH CANDLES AND CONVERSATION

Tell me, my love, where are you leading your flock today?
Where will you rest your sheep at noon?
SONG OF SONGS 1:7

Take time to set the dinner table for two, get a babysitter for the kids if you have children, and maybe even set up a dinner table in your bedroom with candles and good relaxing music or love songs playing.

As you enjoy a meal together, don't talk about your challenges or the frustrating things that happened that day. Instead, focus on your husband. Ask about his day and be a good, loving listener. As you do, you will begin to see him in a whole new way.

3. CONNECT THROUGH TOUCH AND TENDERNESS

Place me like a seal over your heart,
like a seal on your arm.
For love is as strong as death,
its jealousy as enduring as the grave.

Love flashes like fire,
*   the brightest kind of flame.*
SONG OF SONGS 8:6

I once heard a marriage counselor say that a ten-second kiss and hug can begin to heal a marriage. Yet once we're married, we rarely hold our husband's hand while walking or take a moment to look into his eyes and say I love you.

It's time to redefine marriage for ourselves and our children. Take a chance and express your love once again to your man. Even if he doesn't respond at first, continue to love him unconditionally, the way God loves you.

POWER UP WITH PRAYER

Oh, how beautiful you are! How pleasing, my love, how full of delights!
. . . I am my lover's, and he claims me as his own.
SONG OF SONGS 7:6, 10

Dear Lord,
Please renew the love and romance in my marriage.
*   Help me to let go of the little things that keep me from*
expressing love to the man I married. Help me never to take
him for granted and to treat him with love, honor, and
respect. Give him a heart for You, and help him to express
his love to me in a way that draws us closer together. I pray
that we would experience the kind of love that is expressed in
Your Word in the Song of Songs. I pray that You would use
the good and the bad to draw us close to You and close to each
other. Amen.

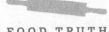

FOOD TRUTH

**No food . . . is as satisfying as
God's love for you.**

Romantic Meal Recipes for Two

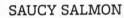

Tell your husband that you love to watch him grill and that flirting in
the kitchen is fun and that . . .

SAUCY SALMON
Serves 2

Ingredients:

¼ teaspoon cinnamon

2 teaspoons honey

2 tablespoons low-sodium soy sauce or Bragg Liquid Aminos

2 tablespoons orange juice

2 salmon fillets (cut thick, about ¾ to 1½ inches)

1 cup cranberry juice cocktail

¾ cup dried cranberries

¼ cup finely chopped onion

1 tablespoon brown sugar

1 teaspoon orange zest

Directions:

1. Soak a cedar grilling plank in water for 3–4 hours.
2. Combine cinnamon, honey, soy sauce or Bragg Liquid Aminos, and orange juice in a shallow dish. Let salmon marinate in mixture for 30 minutes, turning occasionally.
3. Meanwhile, combine cranberry juice cocktail, dried cranberries, onion, brown sugar, and orange zest in medium saucepan. Cook over medium to high heat until the mixture boils, then reduce heat and simmer for 10 minutes. Onions should be tender. Remove sauce from heat and set aside.
4. Heat the grill medium-high for indirect heat. Place the soaked plank on the grill for 3 to 4 minutes or until the plank starts to spit and crackle.
5. Place the salmon skin side down on the hot plank, and place the plank on or under the grill rack. Cook for 20 to 30 minutes, continually basting the salmon with the excess marinade.
6. Place the cooked salmon on plates and drizzle with the cranberry juice cocktail sauce.
7. Have a candlelit dinner with your honey and enjoy some time together!

Recipe tip:

If you and your man like spicier foods, add red pepper flakes to the sauce.

MIDNIGHT CHOCOLATE TRUFFLES

Serves 2

Ingredients:

½ cup heavy whipping cream

8 ounces dark chocolate baking bar, broken into pieces

½ cup finely chopped nuts (optional)

½ cup shredded coconut (optional)

Cocoa powder (optional)

Directions:

1. Line a baking sheet with parchment or wax paper. Heat cream to a gentle boil in a medium-size heavy saucepan. Remove from heat and add the chocolate.
2. Stir until mixture is smooth and chocolate is melted. Refrigerate for 15 to 20 minutes or until slightly thickened.
3. Drop chocolate mixture by rounded measuring teaspoon onto the prepared baking sheet. Refrigerate for 20 minutes.
4. Shape or roll into balls. Coat each chocolate ball with nuts, coconut, or cocoa, if desired.
5. Store in an airtight container in the refrigerator.

Recipe tip:

If the two of you cook these together and feed them to each other, you'll decide that chocolate has never tasted so good!

SWEET BALSAMIC CHICKEN DELIGHT

Serves 2

Ingredients:

2 chicken breasts

½ cup olive oil

½ cup balsamic vinegar

Sea salt and pepper

1 teaspoon ground rosemary

2 cups whole-grain or
   gluten-free pasta

2 tablespoons olive oil

1½ garlic cloves, chopped

1½ tablespoons butter

2 to 4 tablespoons balsamic
   vinegar

1½ teaspoons dried parsley

1 tablespoon onion powder

1 teaspoon raw sugar
   (optional)

Salt and pepper

Directions:

1. Marinate the chicken breasts in olive oil and balsamic vinegar. Sprinkle with sea salt, pepper, and rosemary. Let rest 10 to 15 minutes.

2. In a large saucepan, bring water to a boil and cook pasta according to the package directions. Once it is cooked, drain and set aside.

3. In a nonstick skillet, heat 2 tablespoons olive oil over medium-high heat and add garlic. Cook the chicken breasts until they're done.

4. In the saucepan you used to cook the pasta, melt butter over medium-high heat. Let it cook until it is a nice brown color. Add the pasta and toss to coat. Sprinkle with balsamic vinegar and cook over medium heat for 1 minute. Then add parsley, onion powder, sugar, and salt and pepper to taste. Serve with chicken.

Recipe tip:

There are as many variations of this as there are varieties of pasta.

NOT YOUR MAMA'S MEAT LOAF
Serves 2

Ingredients:

½ medium onion, chopped

1 large garlic clove, minced

½ pound lean ground turkey

½ pound pork sausage

1 tablespoon onion powder

¼ cup brown sugar

1 large egg

¼ cup almond or rice milk

Directions:

1. Preheat oven to 350° and coat a bread loaf pan with nonstick cooking spray.
2. Cook onion over medium heat. Once it is tender, add garlic and cook for 1 to 2 minutes more. Set aside.
3. With your hands, mix the two meats together in a medium bowl. (Do this step with your husband for some kitchen-time flirting!)
4. Add onion powder, brown sugar, egg, and milk to the meat mixture.
5. Add cooked onion and garlic to the mixture.
6. Place meat mixture in the bread pan.
7. Bake uncovered for 1 hour and 15 minutes, and serve.

Recipe tip:

This is delicious with chopped mushrooms added to the mixture!

BEEFY AND LEAFY POCKETS
Serves 2

Ingredients:

½ pound lean ground beef

1½ garlic cloves, minced

½ cup chopped onion

1½ cups chopped fresh spinach

¼ teaspoon ground cumin

⅛ teaspoon salt

6 fresh spinach leaves

1 whole-grain pita bread, halved

2 tablespoons cream cheese, softened

⅛ teaspoon curry powder

Directions:

1. In large nonstick skillet, combine the ground beef, garlic, and onions. Cook over medium heat until mixture is browned, stirring to crumble the beef.
2. Drain off fat, and remove beef mixture from skillet. Clean the skillet, and put beef mixture back in.
3. Add chopped spinach, cumin, and salt. Stir well. Cover and cook over medium heat 3 minutes. Remove from heat.
4. Line each pita half with whole spinach leaves, and spoon ½ cup beef mixture into each.
5. Mix cream cheese with curry powder. Top beef with cream cheese mixture.

Recipe tip:

This is also great with mushrooms! Frying the meat mixture in a little bit of olive oil makes for a crunchier meal.

SWEET CHOCOLATE FONDUE

Serves 2

Ingredients:

8 ounces heavy cream

1 pinch brown sugar

12 ounces dark chocolate, broken into pieces

½ teaspoon vanilla extract

1 pinch sea salt

Strawberries, pineapple, and banana or other fruit of your choice, washed and cut into bite-size pieces

Directions:

1. Warm cream over medium heat until it starts to bubble. Then add brown sugar, dark chocolate, vanilla, and sea salt. Mix until chocolate is melted completely.
2. Pour into heated fondue pot.
3. Using skewers, dip fruit into chocolate and feed bites to each other.

Recipe tip:

This is a very romantic dessert! Get creative with the dipping foods—try pretzels and marshmallows.

OYSTER DELIGHT SOUP WITH ANGEL-HAIR PASTA

Serves 2

Ingredients:

1½ cups whole-grain or gluten-free angel hair pasta

2 green onions, chopped

2 tablespoons melted butter

1 can (16 ounces) unsweetened coconut milk

½ teaspoon red pepper flakes

1 teaspoon sea salt

12-ounce container fresh oysters, undrained

1 tablespoon freshly squeezed or bottled lemon juice

Directions:

1. Cook angel-hair pasta in boiling water, drain, and set aside.
2. In a large pot on medium-high heat, cook green onions in butter.
3. Add coconut milk, red pepper flakes, sea salt, and oysters with liquid to onions and butter. Cook until boiling.
4. Add angel-hair pasta to boiling soup; reduce heat and simmer for 5 minutes. Squeeze lemon juice over soup just before serving.

Recipe tip:

This is really wonderful when you add sliced zucchini, mushrooms, or shrimp! You and your man will love this subtly spicy soup.

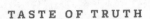

TASTE OF TRUTH

Romantic expressions of love are the perfect gift exchange between a husband and wife.

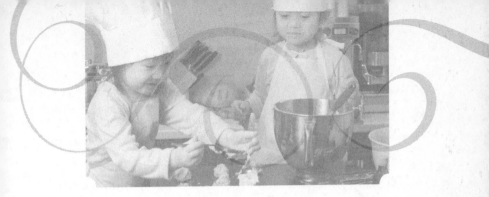

CHAPTER 12

Craving Time with Kids

Healthy Recipes for Kids and Faith Made Real at a Meal

My son, Jake, is now married and has his own little girl, Olive True, our first grandbaby. When I was raising my son, I wanted him to have real faith, but I feared I would not be able to pass that faith on to him. I realize now that faith is not something that can be given away; it is something that, when we live it out, our children will come to crave.

I used to feel guilty for what I considered my shortcomings as a mother; now I realize that God entrusts us with children, and He will cover us when we cannot cover ourselves. He will be faithful to our children even when we fail them. If you're craving to find a way to instill faith in your children, let me first say this to you as a spiritual mom: don't put pressure on yourself; instead, pray and ask God to give your children a heart for Him.

Soul Food

. . . .

We will not hide these truths from our children; we will tell the next generation about the glorious deeds of the LORD, about his power and his mighty wonders.

PSALM 78:4

I always told Jake the truth: while I would let him down, God never would. I am imperfect, but God is perfect. I would not always be there, but God always would be there for him. Today my son knows and loves the Lord in a very real way, not because of my perfection but because of my honesty.

I pray that the following three creative ideas will take the pressure off you and give you joy as you begin to share the love of God with your children.

New Life Recipes

. . . .

1. READ A BIBLE STORY AT THE TABLE AFTER A MEAL

You must love the LORD your God with all your heart, all your soul, and all your strength. And you must commit yourselves wholeheartedly to these commands that I am giving you today. Repeat them again and again to your children. Talk about them when you are at home and when you are on the road, when you are going to bed and when you are getting up.

DEUTERONOMY 6:5-7

Food and faith talk are about as good as it gets when it comes to satisfying both our bodies and souls at mealtime. God talk around the table builds memories and keeps stress levels down.

Keep Bible storybooks in a kitchen cabinet so kids can reach them. Rotate who picks the story to read each night. Once you have read the story, sit for a moment and let your kids share what they learned.

2. WORSHIP IN THE KITCHEN WHILE CLEANING UP

Praise the LORD with melodies on the lyre;
make music for him on the ten-stringed harp.

PSALM 33:2

The Lord wants us to serve one another, yet getting our children to be joyful about cleaning up often becomes more of a chore than the cleaning itself.

Still, you can set the tone and make cleanup more fun. Once you're done with dinner and story time, turn on some upbeat kids' worship songs and turn cleaning into a time of worship. It's hard to complain when worship music is being played, so turn up the volume and watch what happens in your home and in your kids' hearts.

3. LET YOUR CHILDREN PRAY

But Jesus said, "Let the children come to me. Don't stop them! For the Kingdom of Heaven belongs to those who are like these children."

MATTHEW 19:14

Since Jesus wants little children to come to Him, let's teach our precious ones to talk to their heavenly Father in prayer. If they are toddlers, say a prayer one line at a time and let them repeat it after you. Encourage them to talk with God about everything. When prayers they prayed are answered, talk about that with them so they can celebrate God's goodness with you.

POWER UP WITH PRAYER

You are always the same; you will live forever. The children of your people will live in security. Their children's children will thrive in your presence.

PSALM 102:27-28

Dear God,
I lift up my children before You, and I pray that they would
crave You more than anything else. Help me teach them
about You and Your love. Help me not to waste the teachable
moments You give me to share real faith.
I dedicate our mealtimes to nourishing my family's
bodies and souls while we sit and eat together. Help me begin
creative conversations that will draw my children closer to
You and give them hearts to hear who You are. Amen.

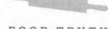

FOOD TRUTH

No food . . . is as enjoyable as being healthy feels.

Recipes for Healthy, Happy Kids

While mealtimes offer an ideal setting to provide soul nourishment to your kids, the kitchen table is also the perfect place to introduce them to great-tasting, healthy foods like the following recipes.

FRUIT POP POPS
Serves 6

Ingredients:
½ cup hulled strawberries

1 banana, cut up

1 mango, cut up

1 cup orange juice

2 apples, peeled, cored, and cut up

2 tablespoons honey, raw sugar, or stevia

Directions:
1. In blender, mix strawberries with banana, and pour mixture into the bottom of each ice pop mold.
2. Blend together the mango and orange juice. Add to the ice pop mold for the second layer.
3. Blend the apples with honey or sugar. Pour into ice pop mold to make the last layer.
4. Put sticks in the molds and place in freezer overnight.

Recipe tip:
Try using pineapple juice instead of orange juice.

PRETTY PUDDING
Serves 4

Ingredients:

3 cups frozen raspberries

2 passion fruits

1 mango

2 dates

1 cup unsweetened applesauce

1 tablespoon canola or sunflower oil

1 tablespoon honey or agave syrup

Directions:

1. In blender, mix together the fruits until smooth.
2. Add applesauce, oil, and sweetener.
3. Blend until smooth and thick. Serve!

Recipe tip:

If your kids love coconut, mix in some shredded coconut after blending for extra texture and flavor.

COCO CRAZY SMOOTHIE

Serves 2

Ingredients:

3 cups coconut milk

1 tablespoon vanilla extract

4 dates or ⅓ cup date sugar or raw sugar

1 tablespoon coconut or grapeseed oil

1½ mangoes

Directions:

1. In blender, mix together all ingredients.
2. Pour and serve.

Recipe tip:

You can substitute banana or pineapple for the mango, depending on what your kids like.

CHOCO SAUCE

Serves 2–4

Ingredients:

2 cups unsweetened applesauce

½ teaspoon vanilla extract

1 tablespoon dark unsweetened cocoa powder

½ cup semisweet chocolate chips

Directions:

1. In blender, mix all ingredients together until smooth.
2. Serve and let your kids enjoy!

Recipe tip:

For extra fun, sprinkle shredded coconut or sliced almonds on top, depending on your kids' preferences.

YUM-YUM NACHOS

Serves 6

Ingredients:

1 cup canned low-fat black beans, drained

1 cooked chicken breast, diced

2 teaspoons freshly squeezed or bottled lime juice

1 clove garlic, minced

1 teaspoon onion powder

7 ounces baked tortilla chips

½ cup shredded cheddar cheese

1 cup low-fat sour cream

Directions:

1. Heat beans in saucepan. Add chicken, lime juice, garlic, and onion powder.
2. Arrange chips on individual plates; spoon beans and chicken mixture over chips. Sprinkle cheese on top, put some sour cream on the side, and serve.

Recipe tip:

You could substitute ground beef or turkey for the chicken. Instead of sour cream, you could add fresh guacamole or salsa on the side.

HEALTHY CHILI CHEESE FRIES

Serves 6

Ingredients:

5 sweet potatoes

Sea salt

Olive oil to drizzle

1 can (15 ounces) red kidney
   beans, drained and
   rinsed

1 cup tomato-based chili
   sauce

2 teaspoons ground cumin

3 cloves garlic, minced

¼ teaspoon black pepper

1 tablespoon Dijon mustard

1½ tablespoons chili powder

1½ cups chicken broth

3 cups chopped cooked
   chicken breast (about
   1¼ pounds)

1 cup shredded cheddar
   cheese

Directions:

1. Preheat oven to 350°.
2. Slice sweet potatoes into strips like french fries. Sprinkle
   with sea salt and olive oil. Bake at 350° for 15 to 20 minutes or
   until crispy.
3. Meanwhile, coat a large saucepan with nonstick cooking spray.
4. Combine kidney beans and chili sauce in the saucepan
   and heat.
5. Add cumin, garlic, pepper, Dijon mustard, chili powder, chicken
   broth, and chicken. Simmer for 10 minutes.
6. Once sweet potato fries and chili are cooked, ladle chili into
   bowls. Sprinkle cheese on top, and add fries on the side. Dip
   fries into chili for healthy chili cheese fries!

Recipe tip:

*This can be a great recipe for adults to enjoy as well. To give it
a spicier kick, add cayenne pepper, green chilies, and jalapeños.*

PIZZA NIGHT

Serves 4–6

Ingredients for pizza crust:

1 teaspoon raw sugar

1½ cups warm water

1 tablespoon active dry yeast

1 tablespoon olive oil

1 teaspoon sea salt

3 cups whole-grain or gluten-free flour, plus additional for
   kneading

Directions for pizza crust:

1. Dissolve sugar in warm water in large mixing bowl. Sprinkle
   yeast over the top. Let stand until foamy, about 10 minutes.
2. Stir olive oil and salt into the yeast mixture. Add 3 cups flour.
3. Place dough on lightly floured surface and knead for about 10
   minutes. Once ball of dough is smooth, place it in an oiled bowl,
   turning the dough until it is evenly coated with oil. Cover with
   a towel and place in a warm place for about 1 hour, until dough
   doubles in size.
4. Place dough onto a lightly floured surface and form into a tight
   ball. Let rise for about 45 minutes, until doubled again. (You can
   divide dough into two smaller balls for two thin-crust pizzas or
   use large ball for one thick-crust pizza.)
5. Preheat oven to 425°. Roll out ball of dough with a rolling
   pin until it won't stretch further. As you shape dough
   into a circle, gently pull the edges outward and rotate the
   crust. Once crust is the desired size, place on a well-oiled
   pizza pan.

Ingredients for pizza sauce:

1 can (6 ounces) tomato paste

¾ cup warm water

2 tablespoons honey

3 tablespoons grated Parmesan cheese

1 teaspoon minced garlic

¾ teaspoon onion powder

¼ teaspoon dried oregano

¼ teaspoon dried thyme

¼ teaspoon dried basil

¼ teaspoon ground black pepper

¼ teaspoon fennel seed

⅛ teaspoon salt (to taste)

Directions for pizza sauce:

1. In a small bowl, mix together all ingredients. Be sure to break up any clumps of cheese.
2. Let sauce sit for 30 minutes to allow flavors to blend.
3. Spread evenly over pizza crust.

Directions for pizza:

1. Once pizza dough has been placed on pizza pan, top with sauce. Then add your choice of cheese, vegetables, and meats.
2. Bake 16 to 20 minutes (depending on thickness) in preheated oven, until the edge of the crust is crisp and golden, and cheese is melted.

Recipe tip:

This will be such fun for your kids! Play restaurant with them, and allow them to get creative with their toppings.

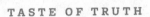

TASTE OF TRUTH

As we teach our children about God, they will begin to teach us through their childlike faith.

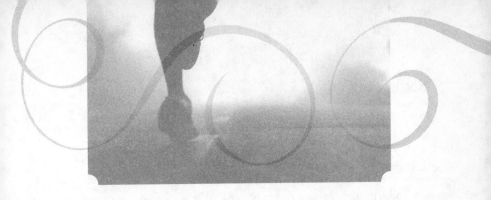

CHAPTER 13

Craving More Energy

Energizing Food and Faith Recipes

WHEN I WAS about to turn forty, I took a personal inventory of all the things I was investing my time in. I then prayed and purposed to delete anything that was draining my strength and energy. Just when I thought I had it all figured out, God gave me and my husband a surprise: I became pregnant with a baby girl.

Now, don't get me wrong, I was excited, but it had been eleven years since I'd had a baby, and at the time I barely had enough energy to make it through each day. Then the reality hit me: when I would be going through menopause, my daughter would be entering her teen years. I looked up toward God and asked, *Where am I going to find the energy to run a ministry and raise a daughter at the same time?*

If I was craving more energy before I discovered I was pregnant, I wondered how I would manage my responsibilities now.

Soul Food

· ·

For I can do everything through Christ, who gives me strength.
PHILIPPIANS 4:13

If we can do all things through Christ, why are we so often exhausted?

To be honest, I think the two things that wear us out most are, first, trying to live in our own strength and, second, attempting to play the junior Holy Spirit. By that I mean we try to control everything in our lives and the lives of those we love. God has wired us to notice situations requiring change and needs that should be met. When He is truly guiding us to take action, He provides the energy and the grace we need to do what we could never do in our own strength. At times, though, we take on burdens He never meant for us to carry.

The truth is, as long as we try to control everything around us, we will feel out of control and overwhelmed. So the first step to gaining energy is to take a deep breath right now and speak these energizing words: "He is God. . . . I am not!" or "I surrender to You, God. Take control and lead me!" God has not called us to burn ourselves out; in fact, one of the things I've learned in my life is that if the devil can't make us bad, his next trick is to make us busy so he can burn us out.

Today my daughter, Emily, is a teenager, and, yes, I do have hot flashes. I find myself desperate every day for more energy and more of God's grace in my life. Maybe you're in a place where you, too, are living out one of God's surprises. Perhaps you're being forced to live a life you never asked for, or maybe you're just sick and tired of being sick and tired. In any event, if you're ready for an energy breakthrough, I encourage you to try three simple practices that have helped give me more energy and renewed passion and joy in spite of the stresses of everyday life.

New Life Recipes

. . . .

1. EXERCISE

Physical training is good, but training for godliness is much better, promising benefits in this life and in the life to come.

    I TIMOTHY 4:8

For years, no matter how many times I was told how good exercise was for me, I dreaded it. I needed an exercise breakthrough. Finally, I decided to make exercise an act of worship. My walks became my worship time and a sacrifice to the Lord. In this way, the Holy Spirit could use my body to do His work through me. Sometimes I put on worship music and danced in my bedroom, just as David danced before the Lord. (Second Samuel 6:14 says David danced in his linen ephod, or priestly garment; I dance with my workout clothes on.) I noticed that as soon as I wasn't exercising for my looks but for my Lord, I began to enjoy exercise for the first time.

How can you find renewed energy through exercise? Make a playlist of your favorite worship songs and choose the type of exercise you enjoy. Instead of thinking of exercise as something you have to do, get up in the morning and praise God that you can move your body and exercise for His glory.

Maybe you have a beautiful place where you can go walking or a friend who will become a prayer partner so you can do prayer walks together. You'll discover that something almost miraculous can happen when all that you do is done for God's glory and not your own!

2. HYDRATE YOUR BODY AND SOUL

But those who drink the water I give will never be thirsty again. It becomes a fresh, bubbling spring within them, giving them eternal life.

    JOHN 4:14

We all want to drink the water Jesus talks about in John 4:14.

He promises that if we drink from His water, we will never thirst again. Many of us are exhausted, I believe, because we are not soaking in the Word that waters our soul. In an attempt to water our thirsty souls, we try artificial faith fixes, which leave us dissatisfied.

Our bodies may also become dehydrated when we don't drink pure water but instead fill ourselves with drinks containing sugar or artificial sweeteners.

Let's try something new. For the next seven mornings, drink a large glass of purified water as you read a short paragraph of Scripture. See how pure water and the Word energize you in a whole new way.

3. ELIMINATE EXCESS IN YOUR LIFE

Therefore, since we are surrounded by such a huge crowd of witnesses to the life of faith, let us strip off every weight that slows us down, especially the sin that so easily trips us up. And let us run with endurance the race God has set before us.

HEBREWS 12:1

For many years, I have spoken at women's conferences. A few years ago, I realized that, the older I got, the more stuff I thought I needed to feel comfortable while on the road. However, every time I came back from a trip my neck and back were out of whack because I dragged heavy luggage through an airport and into a hotel room. Even worse, I never really needed—or used—many of the items I brought!

Many of us have excess activity and busyness that are sucking the life out of us. If you're feeling weighed down, I invite you to take a personal inventory of what you have on your calendar and in your life. Then pray and ask God what He would like you to let go of. Lay that down at His feet and let Him deal with it. If you do this, I believe you will find new strength and the simpler life you crave.

POWER UP WITH PRAYER

But those who trust in the LORD will find new strength. They will soar high on wings like eagles. They will run and not grow weary. They will walk and not faint.

ISAIAH 40:31

Let's make the Word personal and put it into action by praying Isaiah 40:31:

Dear God,
Help me to trust in You, and as I do, give me renewed strength.
Give me eyes to soar above my circumstances and give me a
renewed passion to run in Your strength and not my own. I pray
from this day forward that I will not grow faint but finish
strong. Amen.

FOOD TRUTH

No food . . . is as satisfying as the energy to enjoy life.

Seven Energizing Food Recipes

Now that we've talked about energizing our faith, let's energize our bodies with some delicious meals. I have created seven energizing recipes to help defeat the battle of fatigue once and for all.

Protein is essential to maintaining a healthy body and is an important source of energy. Salad is not only a great way to sneak in our fruit and veggies for the day, but it also helps boost our bodies' antioxidants. The recipes on the following pages are packed full of creative, protein-filled salads or meat entrées that are sure to give you that boost of energy you crave. And they taste amazing!

STEAK SUPREME SALAD
Serves 4

Ingredients for salad:

5 ounces lean steak

2 teaspoons olive oil

1 pinch sea salt

3 to 4 cups spinach, washed
    and dried

1 cup sliced cucumber

8 to 12 strawberries, sliced

1 avocado, peeled and sliced
    (optional)

Ingredients for vinaigrette dressing:

3 tablespoons sherry or red wine vinegar

1 tablespoon Dijon mustard

1 tablespoon honey

2 tablespoons olive oil

1 pinch ground black pepper

Directions:

1. Slice steak into thin strips. Broil or panfry in 2 teaspoons oil; cook meat to your liking. Add sea salt and set meat aside.
2. Combine spinach, cucumber, and strawberries in a salad bowl and toss gently.
3. To make vinaigrette dressing, whisk together sherry or red wine vinegar, Dijon mustard, honey, olive oil, and black pepper in a small bowl.
4. Gently toss the spinach, cucumber, and strawberries with the vinaigrette.
5. Place spinach mixture on individual serving plates. Top with the steak and avocado slices, and serve.

Recipe tip:

Use the vinaigrette dressing for any of your favorite salads. It is always better to make your own than to use a bottled dressing.

FRUIT FIESTA CHICKEN SALAD

Serves 4

Ingredients:

1 head romaine lettuce, torn into bite-size pieces

4 ounces feta or goat cheese, crumbled

1 cup pistachios

¼ cup dried cranberries

1 green apple, peeled, cored, and diced

1 pear, cored and sliced

3 cooked chicken breasts, diced

Freshly squeezed or bottled lemon juice, to taste

¼ cup coconut (optional)

Directions:

1. In a large serving bowl, toss together the romaine lettuce, cheese, pistachios, cranberries, apple, pear, and chicken.
2. Dress the salad with freshly squeezed lemon juice and, if desired, coconut.

CAJUN JUMBO SHRIMP KEBABS

Serves 6

Ingredients for dry rub:

1 teaspoon cinnamon

1 pinch sea salt

½ teaspoon cumin

½ teaspoon ground turmeric

¼ teaspoon paprika

¼ teaspoon pepper

⅛ teaspoon ground cloves

⅛ teaspoon nutmeg

2 teaspoons raw sugar or honey

¼ teaspoon ground ginger (optional)

Ingredients for kebabs:

2 pounds jumbo shrimp, uncooked and cleaned

2 small red onions, peeled and cut into 1-inch wedges

2 red or yellow bell peppers, cleaned and cut into 1-inch squares

¼ cup olive oil

½ teaspoon sea salt

1 pinch black pepper

12 bamboo skewers

Directions:

1. Soak bamboo skewers in water for 30 minutes.
2. Combine the dry rub ingredients in a small bowl, mixing well.
3. Place shrimp into a gallon-size ziplock plastic bag; add the rub mix. Seal the bag and shake it until the shrimp is evenly coated.
4. Place the onions and bell peppers in another gallon-size ziplock plastic bag. Add the olive oil, sea salt, and pepper. Seal the bag and shake to coat the vegetables well.
5. Alternate skewering shrimp and pieces of onion and bell pepper on bamboo skewers.
6. Prepare a charcoal fire or set a gas grill to medium-high, close the lid, and heat until hot—about 10 to 15 minutes.
7. Grill the kebabs about 8 to 10 minutes. Turn them once halfway through cooking time.

ASIAN CABBAGE CRUNCH SALAD

Serves 6

Ingredients for salad:

1 head red cabbage, cut into bite-size pieces

1 head white cabbage, cut into bite-size pieces

2 tablespoons diced cilantro

2 tablespoons green onion

1½ cups diced cooked chicken breast

½ cup sliced almonds

Ingredients for dressing:

1 cup apple cider vinegar

1 cup low-sodium soy sauce or Bragg Liquid Aminos

½ cup honey

Directions:

1. Combine both types of cabbage, cilantro, and green onion.
2. Add chicken and sliced almonds.
3. Mix together the vinegar, soy sauce or Bragg Liquid Aminos, and honey for the dressing.
4. Pour dressing over cabbage and chicken mixture and toss gently.

Recipe tip:

This healthy Asian dressing is a great dip for carrots, celery, or broccoli. You can also use it on any salad you like—get creative!

SUMMERTIME SALAD

Serves 6

Ingredients for salad:

1 seeded and diced cucumber (cut as explained in directions)

7 cups romaine lettuce

1 orange, peeled and sectioned

1 cup thinly sliced radishes

¼ cup shredded raw sweet potato

¼ cup shredded raw beet

¼ cup green onion, thinly sliced

Ingredients for dressing:

2 tablespoons rice or white wine vinegar

2 tablespoons orange juice

1 tablespoon sesame oil

¼ teaspoon sea salt

⅛ teaspoon black pepper

Directions:

1. Cut cucumber into four strips (so that each is in the shape of a dill pickle spear); remove seeds. Dice cucumber strips.
2. Combine the cucumber, lettuce, orange sections, radishes, sweet potato, beet, and green onion in a large bowl.
3. In a smaller bowl, mix vinegar, orange juice, sesame oil, sea salt, and black pepper. Whisk until blended. Pour over salad, tossing gently to coat. Serve immediately.

Recipe tip:

If you prefer fruit to raw sweet potato and beet, you can add diced kiwi, strawberries, and/or blueberries instead.

TUNA ZEST
Serves 1–2

Ingredients:

1 can white albacore tuna in water, drained

½ avocado, smashed

2 teaspoons freshly squeezed or bottled lemon juice, or to taste

Pepper, to taste

¼ cup fresh basil (optional)

Directions:

Mix all ingredients. Eat as is or serve on a slice of whole-grain bread or over a bed of lettuce or spinach.

Recipe tip:

You can also enjoy this tuna dish with whole-grain or gluten-free rice crackers. Served this way, it makes a great dish for your kids!

APPLE CINNAMON CHICKEN AND RICE

Serves 4

Ingredients:

2 cups brown rice

1 tablespoon olive oil

4 skinless, boneless chicken breast halves

Freshly squeezed or bottled lemon juice (optional)

1 tablespoon raw sugar or honey

1 cup unsweetened applesauce

Dash cinnamon

Salt and pepper

Directions:

1. Preheat oven to 350°.
2. Prepare brown rice according to package directions.
3. Warm oil in skillet over medium heat. Add chicken breasts, browning lightly on both sides. (If desired, squeeze lemon juice over chicken as it browns for extra flavor.)
4. Mix the honey into the unsweetened applesauce. Place the browned chicken in a casserole dish, and top evenly with the applesauce and cinnamon. Add pinch of salt and pepper to taste; cover and bake for 35 minutes.
5. Serve with steamed brown rice.

Recipe tip:

This makes a great dinner for the whole family. If you don't want the chicken to be sweet, simply omit the raw sugar or honey.

TASTE OF TRUTH

**You will never regret making time
to renew your strength.**

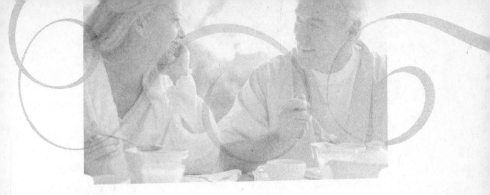

CHAPTER 14

Craving a New Day and a New Beginning

Breakfast Recipes and Blessings to Start Your Day

ONE OF MY FAMILY'S favorite traditions is one of our only consistent rituals. What is it? We have breakfast for dinner once a week. Given our busy schedule, this seems to be the one thing that we can stick to.

There is something so comforting about pancakes and eggs at the dinner hour. We've done it for so many years that even though our grown son is living out of state, his single friends still like to come over and have breakfast for dinner with us old folks.

While this is a fun, long-standing tradition, this chapter centers on the joy that comes from knowing we are offered a new day every morning.

Soul Food

This is the day the LORD has made.
We will rejoice and be glad in it.

PSALM 118:24

175

The greatest thing about a new day is that it offers a new beginning. In that first waking moment, we can decide to worry about tomorrow, live in the regrets of yesterday, or embrace the start of a new beginning.

When you look at each morning as a second chance to live for the Lord and love others well instead of just another day, it will change the way you think and feel. Of course, I know that's easier said than done, especially if you fell asleep the night before feeling regret or pain from your past. With that in mind, here are three New Life Recipes that have helped me break free from starting my day the wrong way. I pray that you, too, will embrace a new way of living . . . one that requires checking into the present day because it's all you have.

New Life Recipes

1. START YOUR DAY WITH PRAISE

> *It is good to give thanks to the LORD,*
> *to sing praises to the Most High.*
> *It is good to proclaim your unfailing love in the morning,*
> *your faithfulness in the evening.*
>
> PSALM 92:1-2

Make a playlist of your favorite praise music, preferably upbeat worship songs that inspire you to live for God. Sing a love song to the Lord on your way to work, or make up your own praise song.

2. START YOUR DAY WITH PRAYER

Pray in the Spirit at all times and on every occasion. Stay alert and be persistent in your prayers for all believers everywhere.

EPHESIANS 6:18

Turn whatever thoughts are on your heart first thing in the morning into a prayer. Your heavenly Father wants to hear from you, and He cares about everything you care about. Don't miss taking the first moments in the morning to connect your heart to His and to bring your concerns and requests to the only one who can do anything about them—God Himself.

3. START YOUR DAY THANKFUL

Fix your thoughts on what is true, and honorable, and right, and pure, and lovely, and admirable. Think about things that are excellent and worthy of praise.

PHILIPPIANS 4:8

As hard as it is to be thankful for a hard day in front of you, let your mind think about anything worthy of praise and any good thing that is coming out of a challenging situation. If you can't find anything worthy of praise, just praise God that He is with you and fighting for you. If you're in a battle, be thankful that you are not alone.

POWER UP WITH PRAYER

*Listen to my cry for help, my King and my God,
     for I pray to no one but you.
Listen to my voice in the morning, LORD.
     Each morning I bring my requests to you and wait expectantly.*

PSALM 5:2-3

*Dear God,
I need the joy You offer on this new day. Give me Your
eyes today; give me Your heart for others. Give me a new
perspective on this day that I may not waste it on worry or
regret. Go before me, Lord, and pave my way today. Amen!*

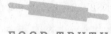

FOOD TRUTH

No food . . . tastes as good as living out God's plan for your day.

Amazing Breakfast Recipes

The way you start your day may very well determine the outcome of the entire day. We often hear that breakfast is the most important meal of the day—and that's true! I have compiled my absolute favorite breakfast recipes to help you start your day off right.

CHOCOLATE CHIP PANCAKES
Serves 4–6

Ingredients:

2 eggs

1 teaspoon vanilla extract

1 cup pancake mix

¾ cup water

1 tablespoon canola or sunflower oil

1 tablespoon cocoa powder

1 tablespoon raw sugar or stevia

½ cup semisweet chocolate chips

Directions:

1. Coat a skillet with nonstick cooking spray and place over low to medium heat.

2. In a medium bowl, mix all ingredients except the chocolate chips until smooth.
3. Pour a half cup of batter into a skillet to form a circle. Sprinkle a small handful of chocolate chips onto the pancake, and let it cook on one side. Then flip.
4. Repeat step 3 until all the batter has been cooked.
5. Serve and enjoy!

Recipe tip:

This also makes a great dessert. Just spread a thin layer of marshmallow creme on top.

BREAKFAST DATE SMOOTHIE

Serves 2–3

Ingredients:

2 cups frozen berries (strawberries, raspberries, and/or blueberries)

1–2 dates

2–3 cups of organic spinach and/or kale

2 tablespoons protein powder

1 cup ice (more if needed)

Directions:

1. Place all ingredients together in blender and mix until smooth.
2. Pour and serve!

Recipe tip:

If you're making this for your kids, don't tell them about the spinach. They won't even taste it, and they will be getting their veggies for the day. If the smoothie doesn't taste sweet enough for you, add some raw sugar or stevia.

MAKEOVER MUFFINS

Serves 8–12

Ingredients:

2 cups whole-grain or gluten-
   free flour

1 cup flaxseed meal

1 cup oat bran

½ cup molasses

½ cup raw sugar or stevia

2 teaspoons baking soda

1 teaspoon baking powder

1 teaspoon sea salt

2 teaspoons cinnamon

¾ cup rice, almond, or
   coconut milk

4 eggs, beaten

1 teaspoon vanilla extract

2 tablespoons canola or
   sunflower oil

1½ cups shredded carrots

2 apples, shredded

1 cup dried blueberries

1 cup pecans, crushed

Directions:

1. Preheat oven to 350° and coat muffin tin with nonstick spray or use paper baking cups.
2. In large bowl, mix together all ingredients (except carrots, fruit, and nuts) until smooth.
3. Add carrots, fruit, and nuts to mixed ingredients.
4. Spoon batter into muffin cups, filling each about halfway full. Bake for 20 to 25 minutes or until golden brown.

Recipe tip:

Take a muffin to work for an afternoon snack or pack some in your kids' lunches. Use decorative paper muffin cups for extra fun!

POACHED PEARS

Serves 4

Ingredients:

½ cup water

4 pears, halved and cored

1 tablespoon freshly squeezed or bottled lime juice

3 tablespoons honey

1½ cups plain nonfat yogurt

Directions:

1. Heat water in skillet and add pears. Cover and cook for 5 to 7 minutes.
2. Remove from heat and add lime juice and honey.
3. Place pears over yogurt and enjoy!

Recipe tip:

For something different, substitute fat-free cottage cheese or oatmeal for the yogurt.

BROCCOLI BACON FRITTATA

Serves 6

Ingredients:

1 cup diced broccoli

¼ cup butter

1 cup sliced fresh mushrooms

1 medium onion, chopped

6 eggs

8 slices turkey bacon, cooked and crumbled

1 small tomato, sliced

4 ounces grated low-fat cheddar cheese

Directions:

1. Place broccoli in a nonstick 10-inch skillet, adding enough water to cover. Bring to a full boil. Cook over medium heat until crisp-tender, 3 to 5 minutes. Drain and place broccoli on a small plate.
2. Melt butter in same skillet. Add mushrooms and onion. Cook over medium heat until tender, about 3 to 4 minutes.
3. Beat eggs together in a bowl until frothy. Add bacon. Pour into skillet and stir gently. Cook on medium heat for 3 to 4 minutes.
4. As eggs set, lift up sides to allow uncooked egg to flow underneath. Arrange broccoli and tomato slices on top. Cover and let cook until eggs are completely set, about 4 to 5 minutes.
5. Sprinkle with cheese and cut into pizzalike wedges. Serve and enjoy!

Recipe tip:

Add chopped spinach for extra greens. You can also replace the turkey bacon with organic ground beef and serve as a dinner casserole.

CINNAMON APPLE MUFFINS

Serves 8–10

Ingredients:

6 tablespoons canola or sunflower oil

1 teaspoon butter

1 cup honey

2 eggs

1½ teaspoons vanilla extract

2 cups whole-grain or gluten-free flour

1 teaspoon cinnamon

½ teaspoon baking soda

½ teaspoon baking powder

½ teaspoon sea salt

⅓ cup unsweetened applesauce

⅔ cup low-fat sour cream

1 Granny Smith apple, peeled, cored, and cut into thin slices

2–4 teaspoons chopped pecans

Honey, for glazing

Directions:

1. Preheat oven to 350° and coat muffin tin with nonstick spray or use paper baking cups.
2. Beat together the oil, butter, and honey with mixer on high speed until mixture is fluffy.
3. Decrease speed and add eggs and vanilla.
4. In a separate bowl, mix the dry ingredients together. Mix half the dry ingredients into the egg mixture; add applesauce and sour cream; then add the rest of the dry ingredients.
5. Spoon batter into muffin cups, filling each about halfway full. Top each cup with apple slices. Sprinkle ¼–½ teaspoon of pecans on each muffin; glaze with honey.
6. Bake on center rack until muffins are golden brown and springy to the touch, about 30 to 35 minutes.

Recipe tip:

This is a great snack or dessert to pack in a lunch box too.

ORIENTAL EGGS

Serves 6

Ingredients:

8 eggs

3 teaspoons low-sodium soy sauce or Bragg Liquid Aminos

1 clove garlic, minced

½ teaspoon toasted sesame oil

½ teaspoon white pepper

½ cup chopped snow peas

½ cup chopped green onion

1½ cups bean sprouts

Directions:

1. Mix eggs, soy sauce or Bragg Liquid Aminos, garlic, sesame oil, and white pepper into a large bowl. Set aside.
2. Coat frying pan with nonstick spray. Cook snow peas and green onion for 2 minutes.
3. Add bean sprouts and cook for 1 minute more.
4. Add egg mixture and cook until firm.

Recipe tip:

You can turn this into a stir-fry for lunch or dinner by adding in 3 cups of cooked brown rice and a meat of your choice.

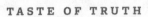

TASTE OF TRUTH

**Every new day is God's gift
of a new beginning.**

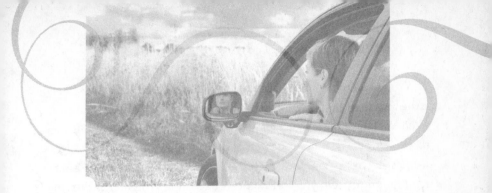

CHAPTER 15

Craving Fresh Adventures

Healthy Food to Go and God Time on the Road

I'VE BEEN ON a lot of airplanes in my life, but one particular flight will forever be engraved on my heart. I remember it as one of my greatest God adventures in the air.

I had been scheduled to be in first class, but the airline had given away my designated seat and put me in the last row by the bathroom. I was assigned to the middle seat between two very large men for the five-hour cross-country flight. As the plane took off, all I could think about was the loss of my first-class seat and how physically exhausted I felt. (They say Jesus can turn water into wine, but He can't turn our whining into anything.) I had such a bad attitude that I decided to try to get some sleep.

But as I started to doze off, I felt the Lord prompting me to ask the man to my left about his daughter. I opened my eyes and looked at the man, thinking, *What if this man doesn't have a daughter?*

I took a chance and asked the man about his girl. When I did, tears welled up in his eyes and he told me how his daughter had gone off to college, only to be raped and become pregnant. He was on his way to get her and take her to get an abortion. As I listened, tears began to flow down my cheeks as well. Still I went ahead and asked a very hard question: "Do you feel that this baby your daughter is carrying deserves a chance at life?" At the time he was in too much pain to answer.

I offered to pray for him and his daughter, even though I had no idea how her situation would turn out. When the plane landed, we said our good-byes. Two years later I was speaking at a conference when a young woman walked up to me holding a little boy. She told me that because of the divine appointment between me and her father on an airplane, she and her dad had talked and prayed, and in the end she'd decided to keep the baby she was holding.

I cried tears of joy and tears of terror as I feared what would have happened if I had allowed my discomfort to keep me from the divine intervention and adventure of faith God wanted me, this man, and his daughter to experience.

Soul Food
. . . .

The Lord went ahead of them. He guided them during the day with a pillar of cloud, and he provided light at night with a pillar of fire. This allowed them to travel by day or by night.

EXODUS 13:21

God put a craving for adventure in the heart of every man and woman. If we don't fulfill our need for adventure with our Lord, we will seek it in the world. His ways and our days need to become one in order for our desire for a faith adventure to be accomplished. Even if we don't have the right attitude, we can be open when the Lord interrupts a disappointing day. When we do, our God will supply the adventure we crave, and daily tasks will become divine appointments.

If you are ready for a God adventure, I invite you to try the buffet of choices below. I am hoping you will taste and see for yourself that the Lord is not only good, He is exciting!

New Life Recipes
. . . .

1. PRAY FOR DIVINE INTERRUPTIONS

Jesus called out to them, "Come, follow me, and I will show you how to fish for people!"

MATTHEW 4:19

One day, Peter started off as a fisherman and ended that same day as one of Jesus' disciples. Look (and pray) for ways to go fishing for a divine interruption today, and you'll find the adventure you're craving!

2. TAKE A JOYRIDE WITH JESUS

You will live in joy and peace. The mountains and hills will burst into song, and the trees of the field will clap their hands!

ISAIAH 55:12

Go for a drive with only one intention: to draw close to the Lord. Pack your Bible, start the praise music, and then stop at a beautiful park. Once you find a quiet place to meet with Him, ask the Lord to become real to you as you read His Word.

3. FUEL YOURSELF WITH THE WORD

In the beginning the Word already existed. The Word was with God, and the Word was God.

JOHN 1:1

A great way to fuel your soul and soothe the frustration caused by traffic jams and time crunches is by listening to Christian books or messages on tape while you drive. Think of long commutes as more time to be inspired by the Word.

POWER UP WITH PRAYER

For God has not given us a spirit of fear and timidity, but of power, love, and self-discipline.

2 TIMOTHY 1:7

> *Dear God,*
> *From this day forward I want to live out my faith as a daily adventure. Please help me not to miss out on time with You. I love You and want more of You every day. Amen.*

FOOD TRUTH

No food . . . is as satisfying as finishing strong.

Food Recipes to Go

The drive-through is not your only (or usually the best) option when you hit the road or plan lunch on workdays. Not only are the following recipes delicious, they will provide you with the fuel you need all afternoon long.

PATTY CAKES

Serves 4

Ingredients:

1½ cups cooked brown rice

2 eggs, beaten

2 tablespoons water

2 teaspoons onion powder

¼ cup shredded sharp cheddar cheese

2 tablespoons olive oil

Directions:

1. Mix all ingredients except olive oil and form into patties.
2. Fry in olive oil in a skillet over medium heat, cooking each patty about 2 to 3 minutes per side.

Recipe tip:

These are perfect to take on a picnic or to the office because they can be eaten hot or cold! You can also add shredded carrots and zucchini to the patties.

YO YO ON THE GO

Serves 1

Ingredients:

⅓ cup almonds

1 cup Greek yogurt

2 teaspoons honey

Directions:

1. Crush the almonds and put them in a to-go bag.
2. When you're ready to eat, sprinkle the almonds over the yogurt and drizzle honey on top.
3. Eat and enjoy!

Recipe tip:

When you're on the go, this handy treat is perfect for an afternoon snack.

BACON-APPLE BITES

Serves 2

Ingredients:

4 turkey bacon strips, cooked

Cheddar cheese slices, cut in 2-inch squares

1 apple, cored and sliced

Directions:

1. Put half a bacon strip and a cheddar cheese square onto an apple slice.
2. Put a toothpick through each stack.
3. Take them with you wherever you go!

Recipe tip:

This is also great with pears. It's the perfect snack to take along on a picnic or pack in a school lunch.

EGGLICIOUS EGG SALAD

Serves 2

Ingredients:

4 eggs, hard boiled and peeled

1½ tablespoons low-fat or Healthy Mayonnaise (see page 21)

1 teaspoon onion powder

1 teaspoon garlic powder

Directions:

1. Mash eggs with a fork.
2. Add mayonnaise, onion powder, and garlic powder. Stir well.
3. This is good served with whole-grain or gluten-free crackers or tortilla chips.

Recipe tip:

This salad will keep in the fridge for three days. Add chopped red onion and bell peppers for color and taste.

MINI ZUCCHINI PIES

Serves 4

Ingredients:

1 tablespoon olive oil	3 eggs
1 onion, chopped	½ cup cheddar cheese, grated
8–12 turkey bacon strips	¼ cup cream cheese
1 large carrot, grated	Salt and pepper, to taste
1 large zucchini, grated	½ cup whole-grain flour

Directions:

1. Preheat oven to 350°.
2. Grease and flour 12 mini muffin tins.
3. Heat the oil in a large pan and sauté the onion. Add the turkey bacon strips and fry to desired crispness. When done, remove bacon from the pan to cool.
4. Add carrot and zucchini to the same pan and cook for about 2 more minutes.
5. Transfer mixture to a bowl to cool. Break up cooled bacon and add to onion, carrot, and zucchini mixture.
6. In another bowl, beat the eggs, cheese, and cream cheese together. Season with salt and pepper as desired.
7. Stir the egg mixture into the cooled onion, carrot, and zucchini mixture. Now stir in the flour.
8. Spoon the mixture into the prepared tins.
9. Bake for 15 to 20 minutes.

Recipe tip:

Perfect for school lunches or a picnic. These muffins can be served hot or cold.

COLD PEA SALAD
Serves 12

Ingredients:

1 bunch green onions, chopped

1 red bell pepper, chopped

5 (12 ounces) cans chickpeas, drained and rinsed

1 bag frozen peas

¼ cup fresh cilantro, chopped

1¼ cups low-fat or Healthy Mayonnaise (see page 21)

1¼ cups plain nonfat yogurt

3 teaspoons ground cumin

3 teaspoons curry powder

1 dash pepper

1 dash onion powder

Directions:

1. Mix onions, bell pepper, chickpeas, peas, and cilantro in a large bowl.
2. Combine mayonnaise, yogurt, cumin, curry powder, pepper, and onion powder in a separate bowl. Mix well and add to vegetables.
3. Serve and enjoy!

Recipe tip:

This is delicious with feta cheese. It's great to take to the office for lunch or send with your kids to school.

SAUTÉED BROCCOLI

Serves 2–3

Ingredients:

1 broccoli head, washed and cut into bite-size pieces

1 cup sliced portobello mushrooms

2 garlic cloves, pressed

1 tablespoon butter

Directions:

1. Place all ingredients in a skillet over low to medium heat. Cook for 10 minutes or until broccoli is tender.
2. Chill and eat.

Recipe tip:

This is another great recipe for lunches or the office. It is best cold but also delicious heated. If you're making this at home for a meal, add chicken for a tasty entrée.

TASTE OF TRUTH

**The real adventure is found
in the unexpected.**

About the Author

SHERI ROSE SHEPHERD is an award-winning author, Bible life coach, and humorist with over one million books sold. Her life experiences help her identify with almost any woman's battle. She grew up in a broken home and was severely overweight as a teen; she also experienced depression, dyslexia, and an eating disorder. Through God's strength, Sheri Rose has become a bestselling author and popular speaker at events nationwide, including Women of Joy and Extraordinary Women. Her weekly video devotions are featured on Bible Gateway. Visit her online at hisprincess.com.

Recipe Index

In *My Beautiful Princess Bible,* Sheri Rose Shepherd helps girls learn what it means to be a daughter of the King of all kings!

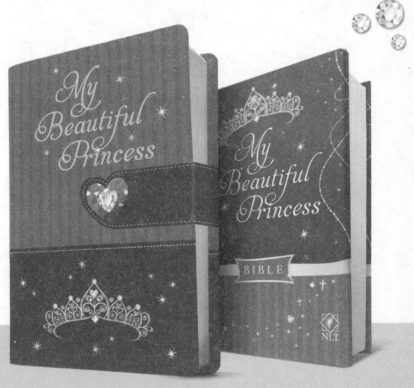

With feature-packed pages, Sheri Rose Shepherd shares a biblical perspective of being God's princesses, and helps girls discover the rich relationship they can have with God through the sacrifice of Jesus on the cross. All of the enhancements in this Bible were specially created to **engage girls in the Word of God** and **instill truth in their hearts** about who God is, how He sees them as His children, and that He has special plans for them!

Available editions:
Padded Hardcover ISBN 978-1-4143-6815-3
Purple Crown LeatherLike (with magnetic closure) ISBN 978-1-4143-7571-9
Deluxe Princess Pink/Purple Royalty LeatherLike (with magnetic closure)
ISBN 978-1-4143-6816-0

CP0561

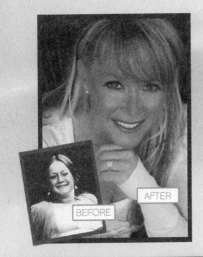